PRAISE FOR GAIL SHEEHY AND
The Silent Passage

"Menopause. In our youth-obsessed culture, the very word is a room-emptier: the pregnancy club is for women a joyous one—the menopause club is one nobody wants to admit she has joined. . . . Gail Sheehy had broken the taboo. She has got notable women talking on the record about the subject. And she has led the way, with candor about herself. . . ."

—Tina Brown

"It is probably the least discussed of the major M words in women's lives. . . . Now Sheehy . . . has set out to end the shame—and the ignorance that fosters it. . . . *THE SILENT PASSAGE* is based on interviews with dozens of medical experts and more than one hundred American women across the socioeconomic spectrum. It offers information on hormone-replacement therapy . . . and urges the millions of baby boomers . . . to view the change as 'the gateway to a second adulthood' rather than a harbinger of the end."

—Kim Hubbard, *People*

"The information is welcome, and Sheehy deserves a cheer for laying on the line what your doctor, your mother, and your best friend won't tell you."

—Amanda Heller, *Boston Sunday Globe*

"Menopause, a topic long avoided by researchers, doctors, the public, and women themselves, is getting new attention, thanks to Gail Sheehy's landmark book and the aging of a baby-boom generation."
—Mary Ann Grossman, *St. Paul Pioneer Press*

"A serious look at the myths and taboos surrounding menopause. . . . *THE SILENT PASSAGE* . . . shot to the No. 1 position in its first week on the [bestseller] list."

—*Entertainment Weekly*

"A compelling discussion about menopause, packed with facts and anecdotes that are right on target for the baby-boom women about to enter the change of life. . . . Laid out eloquently are the facts, the folklore, and the fears. . . ."

—*Kirkus Reviews*

"A call to arms, *THE SILENT PASSAGE* reminds women that they are health consumers, entitled to know a good deal more about their bodies than most know now. Sheehy predicts that as baby boomers begin seeing gynecologists in their later years, they will by sheer force of numbers demand that more attention be paid to menopause, just as they have made similar demands about every other 'passage' in their lives."
—Betty Ann Kevles, *Los Angeles Times*

THE
SILENT
PASSAGE

menopause

GAIL SHEEHY

POCKET BOOKS

New York   London   Toronto   Sydney   Tokyo   Singapore

The author of this book is not a physician and the ideas, procedures, and suggestions in this book are not intended as a substitute for the medical advice of a trained health professional. All matters regarding your health require medical supervision. Consult your physician before adopting the suggestions in this book, as well as about any condition that may require diagnosis or medical attention. The author and publisher disclaim any liability arising directly or indirectly from the use of the book.

 POCKET BOOKS, a division of Simon & Schuster Inc.
1230 Avenue of the Americas, New York, NY 10020

Copyright © 1991, 1992, 1993, 1995, 1998 by G. Merritt Corporation

Published by arrangement with Random House, Inc.

Library of Congress Catalog Card Number: 98–065873

ISBN: 0-671-01774-8

First Pocket Books trade paperback printing June 1998

10 9 8 7 6 5 4 3 2

POCKET and colophon are registered trademarks of
Simon & Schuster Inc.

Cover photo by Carin Riley

Printed in the U.S.A.

Contents

❧

Introduction   xi
Author's Note   xxiii

The Need to Know and the Fear of Knowing   1

"You're Not Old Enough"   14
When You Least Expect It   20
Cinderella Hits Menopause   28
Deal or Deny?   39
Mother Doesn't Always Know Best   46
Monkeying with Evolution   50
Whose Menopause Is It Anyway?   56
Is There a Male Menopause?   60

vii

Contents

Menopause in the Workplace   65

Human Resource Professionals
on the Front Lines   72

The Perimenopause Panic   77

Early Signs   84
Best Defenses   87
Silent Changes   90
Dancing Around Depression   94
From the Pits to the Peak   100
"Stress Menopause"   104
Menopause Moms   107
Sex and the Change-of-Life Lover   111
The "Who Needs Men?" Argument   116
Sex and the Single Woman
of a Certain Age   119
Testosterone for Women   122
Vaginal Estrogen   126
Educating Your Man   128

Estrogen and Brainpower   133

Has Anyone Seen My Memory?   138
Growing and Regenerating Brain   145
Where to Find Your Memory   147

Contents

The Menopause Gateway 151

Partnering Yourself Through a Natural
Menopause 159
The Hidden Thieves 168
The Cheating Heart 170
Embezzled Bone 177
Dangerous Breasts 183
What Is Your Lifetime
Estrogen Budget? 190

Hormone Replacement
Therapy:
Should I or Shouldn't I? 195

Best Bets 200
Outgrown Worries 204
Asking the Right Questions 208
The Weight-Gain Conundrum 216
Do I Have to Stay on Hormones Forever? 220
A New Regimen for Postmenopause 222
New Frontiers in Treatment 224
Making Your Choice 228

Contents

Cultural Catch-Up 231

Doctors Coming out of the Dark Ages 233
The Hysterectomy Trap 238
The "What About Me?" Syndrome 244
Across Color, Class, and Culture Lines 248

Postmenopause and Coalescence 255

Extra-Sexual Passions 262
Wisewoman Power 267
Emptying and Refilling 270

Postscript 275

Index 281

Introduction

As I sit down to update the fourth edition of this book, I am still amazed by the crying need for it. Not just for myself but for other women. A new generation of women—baby boomers—may be reinventing the taboo around menopause.

A group of women in their middling forties left their corporate cubicles early one Friday afternoon to celebrate the forty-fifth birthday of their supervisor. Judging by the knees poking out from their miniskirts to the flex of their well-defined triceps when they reached for the sugar substitute, they were clearly fit, confident and conspicuously conscious of their youthfulness. One sentence from their supervisor shattered all that.

"I can't sleep. I have fevers at night. I keep forgetting my friends' phone numbers. Is this what forty-five feels like or do I have a brain tumor?"

The boldest of the group dared to say, "Well, maybe you're starting menopause."

"I'd rather have a brain tumor."

It was as though a nine-hundred-pound gorilla had just jumped on the table. No one knew what to say. Finally, the boss laughed it off: "Maybe I'm pregnant."

A coworker jumped in, "That's what you get for looking so great at your age, birthday girl!"

Another added, "Anyway, what's the big deal about menopause? We all know our bodies so well, we'll know how to handle it. Your period ends, you have a few hot flashes and that's it."

"Yeah, right," said another co-worker, impatient to change the subject. "Who wants to share a dessert?"

The gorilla was summarily pushed off the table.

But leaving the lunch the birthday "girl" thought about making an appointment with her gynecologist. Now, if she could only remember her name.

Like many women of her age, this hard-working wife and mother had a grab bag of questions about the next stage of her life. They had accumulated from vague conversations with her mother, a few horror stories from friends, and articles only half-digested— articles that discussed heart disease and bone loss, or the risk-benefit ratio of using hormones versus brewing teas made of unpronounceable barks and herbs. But what was really on her mind were the more superficially frightening signs that something was changing: thinning skin, waning sex drive, scattered focus and forgetting people's names. Was this the dreaded downhill slide? Would it always be this way? And there were more questions:

What is perimenopause anyway? What are the

signs? Is there anything you can do about it ahead of time?

Should you start on hormones right away?

What is the real risk of breast cancer?

Does menopause cause permanent memory loss?

What are the alternatives to conventional therapy?

Do alternative therapies really protect your heart and bones?

What nutritional aspects need to be considered?

What's the downside of using hormone therapy over a lifetime?

When I hear stories like this, it reminds me of the constant need to expand our consciousness about this silent passage. It is not the inevitable harbinger of a downhill slide. It is potentially a bridge from the choppy years of family and career-building, when one never seems able to balance all the demands, to a more serene stage of life where, buoyed by greater self-knowledge and skill in handling others, a woman can find her voice and extend her reach into realms never imagined when she was blindsided by the vanities of youth. But the bridge usually does cross over turbulent waters.

I remember only too well my own ignorance. About pregnancy we are taught everything one could want to know. I remember readily finding books on natural childbirth in the library and teaching myself the breathing exercises, so that by the time I went into labor I felt fully prepared. I went into menopause knowing nothing—not even that I was in it. Like so many women who have always enjoyed good health and who prided themselves, upon reaching their mid-forties, on having achieved a fair degree of control over their lives, I was sure I would just "sail right through it." Instead, I veered off course, lost some of the wind in my sails, and almost capsized.

But in trying to learn or to talk about menopause, I found myself up against a powerful and mysterious taboo. My friends were adrift in the same fog. We couldn't help one another because none of us knew enough. Or we didn't want to know. It was as though we had been living with a conspiracy of silence.

After some thought I decided to break the silence and go public with my own, not uncommon, experience and eventually found other well-known women willing to do the same. Initially, Tina Brown, then the editor of *Vanity Fair,* took the bold step of publishing my material in a 1991 magazine article. The electrifying response was the impetus to expand my research and interviews into a book.

When *The Silent Passage* was first published in America in May 1992, it touched a nerve much deeper than I had imagined. From my explorations in America, Canada, and Europe I had some inkling of how backward we are in basic scientific research on a condition that goes back to prehistory. Menopause is not some new environmental toxin, after all. But I had no concept of the shocking breadth of fear, shame, and denial that women would discover among themselves.

Introduction

When I appeared on *Oprah,* her producer admitted that they had had an easier time booking guests to talk about murdering their spouses than about menopause. With tongue in cheek I suggested, "Why not have them both on the same show? They're probably the same people."

By the mid-Nineties, American women wielded enough influence as scientists, physicians, nurses, legislators, journalists, and magazine editors that when they threw their weight behind opening up this subject in Congress and in the media, a huge wave of interest in menopause spread throughout society. We all seem to have discovered at the same time our appalling lack of basic knowledge about this universal female transition. More pointedly, we had almost no hard data on the safety and efficacy of the hormone therapy routinely prescribed to millions of women—perhaps the largest *un*controlled clinical trial in the history of medicine.

But we are catching up fast. Thousands of women's health clinics have sprouted across the U.S. The demographics are undeniable:

- Every day, three thousand five hundred new American women enter menopause.
- By the year 2000, fifty million American women will be in or beyond menopause.
- Women between forty and sixty are the fastest-growing segment of the American population. In European countries the population is aging even more quickly.

Sheer numbers may at last confer normalcy on this predictable passage. And these demographics drastically alter the politics of menopause. Women's health activists have acquired such a large constituency among this not-so-silent majority of midlife women that international drug companies and federal regulatory agencies now must listen to them. As an original member of the advisory board to the Women's Health Initiative, the largest clinical study of women's health in American history, I was privileged to serve with some of the most prominent physicians and scientific researchers in the field of menopause. Even though the earliest results from WHI will not be available until the year 2000, the probing questions generated by this group have already helped to raise the level of awareness within the scientific establishment.

Yet even today, nearing the end of the century, a new generation is discovering its ignorance.

Author Anna Quindlen, forty-five, one of the more savvy voices of the boomer generation, wrote of her own experience in a *New York Times* column, "I should know as much about menopause from talking and listening as I do about pregnancy. But I don't. That is why, when I began to wake bolt upright in the middle of the night and started forgetting the names of my children, I initially thought I was losing my mind."

Boomer women may have an even harder time dealing with menopause than women of previous generations. Their older sisters in the "Silent Generation" and their mothers in the WWII generation simply didn't talk about it at all; their mental engines were expected to slow down, many fewer of them held responsible jobs, and most accepted their invisibility. They became amiable grandmothers or

continued to hold center stage by becoming terrifying
viragos.

Menopause used to shout "middle age." But boomers simply aren't having middle age. Youth is intrinsic
to their identity. And, in fact, boomers are the benefi-
ciaries of a revolution in the life cycle. As I described
in my recent book, *New Passages: Mapping Your Life
Across Time,* in the space of one short generation the
whole shape of the adult life cycle has been funda-
mentally altered. The territory of the fifties, sixties,
and beyond is changing so radically, it now opens up
whole new passages leading to stages of life that are
nothing like what our parents or grandparents experienced.

Cathy Dwyer, president of Revlon, is one among a
new generation of female executives who refutes the
stereotype. Working largely with a staff of thirty- to
forty-two-year-old females, she queried her employees
about their thoughts on what it means to be a fifty-
year-old woman. As expected, she got the same old
tired answers. She then turned to her staff, this
slender, fit, pixie-haired woman with skin as fresh as a
peeled pear, and said, "Well, you're looking at a forty-
eight-year-old one!" Her young staffers were stunned.
The numbers didn't compute with their outdated
images.

Fifty is what forty used to be.

One of the more striking developments is that
women are entering the long menopausal passage
earlier today, as much as five years earlier. It is not
uncommon for the first signs and symptoms to register in the early-to-mid forties, even though a woman
may not officially cross into menopause—defined as

being without menstrual periods for one year—until she is fifty or fifty-one.

No matter what generation we belong to or how much information is available, each woman entering this passage has to reinvent the wheel.

"Just about everybody has a preconceived idea of what menopause will be like and when it will occur," says Dr. Howard Zacur, director of the Johns Hopkins Estrogen Consultation Service. "The actual reality may be so very different, that the association with menopause isn't made."

This edition of *The Silent Passage* has been completely revised to reflect the many exciting developments that have taken place over the last several years. Issues of intense interest to women and health professionals have been fully reported and fleshed out in the form of new chapters:

The Perimenopause Panic describes in detail the most confusing and symptomatic phase of this long passage. To allay the panic of younger women, this chapter prepares them to recognize and relieve the *short-term* symptoms, and make them aware of how to protect against the silent, *long-term* assaults to their health and well-being.

Menopause in the Workplace explores the attitudes and obstacles that career women are discovering in the many work situations where menopause is still denied or misunderstood. The special strengths of the postmenopausal woman employee or executive are traced back to ancient cultures, where older women were central to survival of the tribe.

Today, women entering the age of menopause are likely to be holding down responsible jobs and to have children still at home. They have been the take-charge generation. Those in demanding careers usually accelerate their efforts between age forty-five and fifty, when a woman either "makes it" into the top ranks or levels off. This acceleration in the workplace is likely to coincide with the body's "pause" for menopause. As working women begin to experience embarrassing symptoms like hot flashes and erratic bleeding, they are demanding that more attention be paid to menopause. It is becoming a public health issue.

Estrogen and Brainpower brings out of hiding the latest evidence that estrogen has a critical effect on memory and concentration—in both men and women. A new generation of boomer women are demanding to know what to do about it.

New Frontiers in Treatment is an unbiased critique of the much-publicized new class of drugs—SERMS—known as "designer estrogens." A promising possibility for women who are hypersensitive to progesterone is discussed.

We are no longer alone in the silent passage. We don't have to suffer the shame and depression that overtook many of our mothers. Today there is a whole new way to think about the Change of Life.

You can plan for your menopause the way pregnancies can be planned.

Let that idea sink in as you read this book. You can start planning by talking candidly with mentors who are older than you, by searching out information in books and magazines, and by attending the women's health conferences that are now routinely held in most communities. You can also begin to establish a lifelong relationship with a doctor who has a genuine interest in mature women and who understands the necessity of treating them as partners.

Another new concept that permeates this revised edition is the idea of *customizing* your approach to menopause. Menopause is as individual as a thumbprint. No two women experience it alike. Some wonder what all the fuss is about, since they scarcely register any physical change. Others are bombarded by so many inexplicable symptoms, they wonder if they're going crazy. And many are misdiagnosed— sent off to see a neurologist or a cardiologist or a psychiatrist. Such blind alleys can be avoided with a little effort.

Each one of us has to examine our own thumbprint—that is, collect the information about our family's health history and consciously prepare ourselves for menopause. This edition of *The Silent Passage* offers a much fuller and more sophisticated set of natural remedies and practices for partnering yourself through perimenopause to postmenopause. (See section "The Menopause Gateway.") Each woman will have to decide for herself whether or not the benefits of hormone therapy are worth the risks in her case. (See section "Hormone Replacement Therapy: Should I or Shouldn't I?") But once she has her own health profile clearly in mind, if she does decide to use hormones, a specific hormonal replacement regimen can be designed to meet her health needs. Doctors can adjust doses and regimens for each woman to suit the reactions of her body. But we can't expect doctors to take all the responsibility for customizing treatment. We have to educate ourselves to be informed partners.

The important point is that women in the Change today have choices; they need not follow anybody's manifesto or accept a one-size-fits-all prescription. This book is meant to empower women by informing them of the many different ways they can protect their bodies and promote their mental well-being through menopause and beyond, so they can look forward to finding passions and purposes apart from being vessels of reproduction.

You can become master of your menopause.

Some of the stories herein are cautionary tales of embittered or self-deluding women. And some are snapshots of women who have given themselves every chance to live out the length of their days in full, rich ways. I hope the stories of the women in this book will act as a catalyst for honest conversations about the menopausal experience between mothers and daughters, wives and husbands, women and their doctors.

This book, then, has three purposes: First, to shatter the myths about menopause. Second, to emphasize that menopause is a health issue, and to coach women on how to educate themselves, their doctors, and the men in their lives. And finally, most important, I want to leave readers with another way to think about this stage of a woman's life—what I call our Second Adulthood.

I am happy to report that since the original publication of this book, a new camaraderie has developed among women who are full of juice, humor, and determination to turn this passage into a celebration. They are inventing fiftieth birthday rituals and forming "fan clubs" to share experiences, swap tips, and develop directories of doctors who are knowledgeable, or at least educable, about menopause. In many ways, there has never been a better time in history to pass through menopause.

In that spirit, California women asked me to pass along this motto, which is being hung up on more and more office walls:

WOMEN DON'T HAVE HOT FLASHES
THEY HAVE POWER SURGES!

—G.S.

Author's Note

A further word on method. In my research, I sought out women from all social levels and races and regions. I conducted intimate group interviews, as well as collected individual life histories, in places as dissimilar as Eugene, Oregon; Rochester, New York; Louisville, Kentucky; downtown Los Angeles and Beverly Hills in California; Queens and Manhattan in New York; as well as talking to women online. Participants included privileged women and low-income government workers, women of color and polite white suburbanites, early-forties women anticipating the Change and women in their sixties who could look back on it with some perspective. I interviewed over one hundred women in various stages of menopause and have since talked with thousands more as lectures have taken me around the country.

More detailed medical information was also necessary to raise awareness among women as health consumers. I freely crossed disciplines, reaching beyond the obvious medical practitioners—gynecologists, breast surgeons, and internists—to endocrinologists, who study the hard science of hormones, and epidemiologists, who measure all the factors contributing to a condition like menopause in large populations. Additional light was shed on this complex life transition by interviews with research physiologists, neuroscientists, psychologists, psychiatrists, and gerontologists; and practical approaches to coping with it were suggested by nutritionists and Chinese medicine doctors. For a larger historical and evolutionary perspective I consulted scholars in sociology and anthropology, historians, and primate researchers. I have interviewed well over one hundred experts.

But I have not been altogether alone in my explorations. Dr. Patricia Allen, a gifted obstetrician-gynecologist in private practice in Manhattan and on the staff at New York Hospital-Cornell Medical Center, took an interest in my efforts—both as my personal doctor and as a professional committed to expanding health education for women. She introduced me to top specialists in related fields and took to the trenches with me to listen in on some of the group interviews. It is an ongoing journey of discovery for both Dr. Allen and myself, as we constantly compare notes, reevaluate conventional wisdom, and probe new scientific findings for revised editions of *The Silent Passage*.

We have now become full partners in launching the New York Menopause Research Foundation. We are most fortunate in being associated with the nationally acclaimed Strang Cancer Prevention Center in New York, headed by a member of our board of directors, Dr. Michael Osborne, a prominent breast cancer surgeon and research scientist. Given the ever-expanding number of women approaching this passage who want solid research on which to make informed decisions about how to manage their menopause, and an ever-growing number of basic scientists, clinical investigators, and pioneering physicians who are addressing their concerns, Dr. Allen and I are very excited about adding our efforts to the activist momentum. The New York Menopause Research Foundation will initiate and support small research projects as far-ranging as menopause in the workplace to the effects of estrogen on cognition. Another goal of the foundation is to be a watchdog for women. We will react, in a timely and skeptical fashion, to the hype surrounding launches of all new products, alternative as well as mainstream, with the intention of protecting women from the understandable wish to get something for nothing.

My thanks go to Dr. William J. Ledger, professor and chairman of Obstetrics and Gynecology at New York Hospital-Cornell Medical Center, to Dr. Jamie Grifo, a new-generation gynecologist and research scientist, and to Dr. Robert Lindsay, a leading research endocrinologist in the field of menopause medicine and practitioner at Helen Hayes Bone Center, all of whom read the manuscript and added valuable suggestions and refinements. Trudy Bush, Ph.D., a University of Maryland epidemiologist and one of the principal investigators in the PEPI study of hormone replacement therapy, has kept me well-informed of the implications of this important research. The North American Menopause Society, including Pamela P. Boggs, Director of Education and Development, has also provided me with cutting-edge research.

For this revised edition I have turned for further expertise to members of the board of the New York Menopause Center: Dr. Michael Osborne, director of the Strang-Cornell Breast Center and chief of the

Breast Service at The New York Hospital-Cornell Medical Center; Dr. David Zackson, endocrinologist and nephrologist, director of calcium metabolism in the Division of Endocrinology at the New York Hospital; and Dr. Louis J. Arone, clinical associate professor of medicine at Cornell University Medical College.

In Britain, Dr. Malcolm Whitehead, director of the Menopause Clinic of Kings College Hospital, London, and president of the International Menopause Society, together with his senior research fellow, Dr. Mike Ellerington, were mines of information on the state of research and treatment in the U.K. Dr. Denning Cai, a Chinese medicine doctor in Tarzana, California, and Dr. Shyam Singha, a world-renowned homeopathic practitioner and teacher in England, added a nontraditional treatment perspective.

It has been my privilege to work with one of this country's most distinguished editors, Robert Loomis, at Random House. For this new revised edition I enjoyed the fresh perspective of Nancy Miller, senior editor at Pocket Books, a baby boomer who represents a whole new generation approaching menopause with a whole new set of taboos. It has also been my good fortune to have the tireless research support of Leora Tanenbaum and the further quick-witted research and editorial contributions of Jane Centofante and Rebecca Donner.

The women who gallantly contributed their personal stories to this book are also my partners. Some of their names and backgrounds had to be altered, but others offered their real names. To each one I offer thanks for striking one more small blow for normalization of a proud stage of life.

The
Need to Know
and the Fear
of Knowing

$\mathcal{W}$e think of ourselves as so liberated today that we can talk about anything. In an Oprahfied age people will tell strangers about their abortions or alcoholism, even declare on national television that they are dying of AIDS, yet just let a man suggest to his sleepless, perspiring, weepy wife that her uncharacteristic moods and symptoms might have something to do with menopause and he's bound to get a blanket denial: "What are you talking about! I'm too young!"

Menopause may be the last taboo. The first friend to whom I ever mentioned the subject was a sultry-looking woman of fifty. She had always prided herself on her appearance and gained much of her status from creatively supporting her husband, a successful author who looks somewhat younger than she. I asked if she had ever talked with anyone about menopause.

"No. And I don't want to."

"Women don't bring up the subject around you?"

"One friend did," she said sourly. "I haven't seen her since."

Another friend, a public television producer whose natural temperament is appallingly calm, recalled with rueful laughter her first sign of the Change of Life. She was seated between two titans of industry at a high-protocol Park Avenue dinner party, the kind where the place cards look like tracings from the *Book of Kells,* and she was feeling particularly confident and pretty in her new black designer suit with its flattering white satin collar, when out of the blue a droplet of something hit her collar. Then another drop. What the—was the help dribbling wine? Could there be a leaky ceiling under all that gorgeous boiserie? Suddenly she noticed her husband's gaze turn to alarm from across the table: What horrible thing was happening to her? She put a hand to her face. Her forehead was wet as a swamp.

Oh no, said her eyes, *not me!* as the moisture began running in rivulets down her face and slipping off her chin—*plop*—onto her pearly satin collar. *Should I pick up the white linen napkin and wipe my forehead?* She reached for the five-hundred-threads-per-inch napery, hesitated—*no, all the makeup will come off on the damn napkin*—when a few more plops fell into her décolletage. Frantic, she began dabbing at her face. Trying to pretend it wasn't happening, she turned to her dinner partner and began smiling and mopping, chatting and fanning, laughing at his jokes and dabbing, trying to keep up her end of the conversation while she wanted nothing more in this world than to disappear into the kitchen and tear off her clothes and open the freezer door—never mind that it was February—and just *stand there.*

She and her husband have since had the Thermostat Wars usual in menopausal households—"It's freezing in here!" "No, it's boiling." "Did you turn the thermostat below fifty again?" "Oh, why don't you just get flannel pajamas!" But the producer is one of the lucky ones: She has had no other indicators beyond hot flashes that she is passing into another stage of life.

It happens to every woman. Pregnancy we can choose to go through or not. With menopause there is no choice. It happens to teachers and discount store clerks and dental hygienists, who nonetheless have to function in public, on their feet, every day. It happens to Navy pilots and gray-haired graduate students and former Olympic athletes, who are accustomed to demanding the highest physical and mental performance from themselves. It happens to women of color, to women in the home, it happens even in Hollywood. Gorgeous Goldie, Whoopi Goldberg, Susan Sarandon, Diane Keaton, Jessica Lange, and Candy Bergen, too, must deal with menopause. These women are hardly over the hill. In fact, they are more potent than ever.

But they never mention the big M.

The central myth is that menopause is a time in a woman's life when she goes batty for a few years— subject to wild rages and deep depressions—and after it she mourns her lost youth and fades into the woodwork. In truth, menopause is a bridge to the most vital and liberated period in a woman's life. Certainly hormones have a powerful effect on our physical life and our mood, just as hormones underlie male aggression and affect potency as men age. During the passage through menopause, when hormones are spiking and falling a few times every day, or possibly within an hour, many women do experience waves of fatigue and bouts of the blues. But that is very different from clinical depression. And most important, it is temporary.

In fact, women in their fifties, once through menopause, have the lowest rates of clinical depression compared to women at any other stage of life. Depression actually subsides with age for women.

Ironically, the people who are the most evasive and unsympathetic about menopause tend to be women in their forties. Slouching toward the bridge to that unknown and frightening new territory of "postmenopausal woman," they may become "menophobic." Their own resistance to identifying with the stage of life beyond reproductivity is sometimes expressed in an uncharacteristic intolerance of their own friends.

A thirty-nine-year-old Chicago woman moved to a new city the year her premature menopause came on. Although she made new friends quickly, they began to shun her as soon as she mentioned physical signs associated with the Change. The ostracized woman struggled through five years with a large fibroid cyst and digestive problems before her friends and doctors acknowledged the source of her difficulties.

"I clearly remember not being sympathetic," recalled one of her friends with considerable regret. Others of the woman's friends remembered their impatience. "We'd talk about her among ourselves: 'She's complaining about hot flashes and stomach problems again this week. Why doesn't she just get over it?' We never really said, 'She's suffering.' We certainly never mentioned the possibility of menopause. And here we are, *women."*

"Women can be the worst," acknowledged her best friend.

The formerly shunned woman now realizes, "People wouldn't relate my problems to menopause because that would automatically classify them as old."

Menopause must be one of the most misunderstood passages in a woman's life. One study showed that two-thirds of all American women say nothing to anybody as they approach what may be a distressing and even fearsome Change. But who can blame us? Menopause is inextricably linked with middle age, and in the youth-oriented societies of North America and Europe even the mention of middle age has a stigma about it. Shame, fear, and misinformation are the vague demons that have kept us silent about a passage that could not be more universal among females. The most common fears are: *I'll lose my looks, I'll lose my sex appeal, I'll get depressed, I'll become invisible.* We don't have to lose any of these things. Yet the obvious sources of information and comfort—mothers, doctors, academics—have shied away from the subject. All that is changing as the subject of menopause becomes part of our public conversation.

Today fifty is the apex of the female life cycle. And menopause is more properly seen as the gateway to a Second Adulthood, a series of stages never before part of the predictable life cycle for other than the very long-lived.

If forty-five is the old age of youth, fifty is the youth of a woman's Second Adulthood. In fact, we can

anticipate at least as many years of life after menopause as we have already lived as reproductive wom-
en. You don't believe it? Consider. Most women begin
menstruating around thirteen and begin stopping at
around forty-eight—remaining defined, and confined, to some degree by their procreative abilities for
thirty-five years. The life expectancy of an average
woman who lives to age fifty in the U.S. or U.K. is
now eighty-one. (A man of fifty can expect to live until
seventy-six.) So, from the time she reaches perimenopause, the average woman has thirty-three more
years.

The projected life span of the current generation of
women now hitting fifty in the U.S. is beyond anything known by the human species. They can expect
to live routinely into their eighties and nineties. Here
is the most stunning statistic, affirmed by Kenneth
Manton, research professor of demographic studies at
Duke University.

*A healthy, fifty-year-old American woman who
does not succumb to heart disease or cancer can
expect to see her* ninety-second birthday.

Whoever prepared us for the possibility that we
might live long enough to forget the name of our first
husband?

Since there has been virtually no period in the
history of the human species when evolution has
favored postmenopausal females, we shall have to
favor ourselves. We shall *have to* intervene—medi-
cally, hormonally, psychologically, spiritually—because we cannot assume that aging will go smoothly.
Evolution didn't provide for it.

8

The main point is that we are living longer lives than ever before. But my impression from talking to thousands of women all over America and Europe is that this new perspective—only milliseconds old in evolutionary terms—has not caught up with most people.

Women today often believe they are well-informed about menopause. But the majority of women regard menopause as a short-term event and do not connect it with long-term health problems in postmenopausal life, such as heart disease, osteoporosis, or cancer. Less than half the women in a recent Gallup survey related the Change to these important issues, and more than one in four did not see a doctor at all, because they felt their symptoms were a natural part of menopause.

A keen social observer, British novelist Fay Weldon, points to the psychology of these women: "They'd on the whole rather not know—for if we don't know, it doesn't matter." But it does matter. It matters whether or not a woman in her sixties finds it painful to walk or even bend as a result of osteoporosis. It matters when a woman in her fifties has a heart attack. It matters that women look these possibilities in the eye, because the way in which they approach menopause will affect the risk of their suffering from these diseases. Naturally, parts of our bodies are going to break down with the aging process. Since many of us can expect to live into our eighties or nineties—whether we wish to or not— do we want to have bones and hearts that break down while the rest of us keeps going?

Menopause must be approached today with a different attitude, one that is self-valuing, rather than self-deprecating. Making the effort to change eating, smoking, sleeping, and exercise habits, or taking the time to experiment with hormone replacement or homeopathic practices to help rebalance the body around its new hormonal state, is not an issue of vanity, or attracting men, or succumbing to Western culture's preoccupation with youth. It is an issue of physical and mental *health*.

It is time to render normalcy to a normal physical process that ushers in the youth of our Second Adulthood. This is a passage as momentous as the rite of passage into adolescence. Indeed, the menopausal passage is almost the mirror image of the transition to adolescence for females, and it will take just as many years. Jolted into menstruating at twelve or thirteen—remember?—it took five years or more for our bodies to adjust to our uniquely altered chemistry, while our minds struggled to incorporate our new self-image. So, too, must we readjust to *not* menstruating.

Just as we were apprehensive as eleven-year-olds, standing on the doorsill of childhood, about to be pushed out into the unknown turbulence of puberty, so are we naturally nervous at the approach of menopause, about letting go of aspects of femininity that have defined us. We become more acutely aware of health, appearance, economic security, and the harbingers of mortality.

Another reason for the fear inspired by the prospect of menopause is the assumption that it takes place at a single point in time. Women are very frightened that at age forty-nine, all these things they've read about—heart disease, osteoporosis, vaginal atrophy—will happen at once. No distinction is made between women's lives at fifty and at seventy. We would never do this with men.

It is important, then, to distinguish among the various phases of the long menopausal passage. Archie Bunker probably spoke for many impatient husbands when he pressed his long-suffering wife in a 1972 episode of *All in the Family.*

ARCHIE: Edith, if you're gonna have a change of life, you gotta do it right now. I'm gonna give you just thirty seconds. Now come on, CHANGE!

EDITH: Can I finish my soup first?

Linda Lavin, in her role as Edie Kurland on ABC's series, *Room for Two,* opened the window to this subject on prime time TV in 1993 when she did an episode entitled "A Pause for Menopause." From *Roseanne* to *Murphy Brown,* sitcoms are beginning to reverberate with menopause humor. Women are writing novels and producing films that encompass the rite of passage that transforms them from childbearers to wisewomen.

In the hugely popular film *First Wives Club,* three college friends are reunited at the age of forty-six at the funeral of a friend. They discover they have all been left by their husbands for younger women and set out to get revenge by ruining their exes financially. One of the three is Goldie Hawn who plays an actress. The husband of Hawn's character has stolen her business. When she charges into her ex's office to confiscate his possessions, he wheedles and gets nowhere. Finally, he throws his hands up in the air and strikes back where he knows she will be vulnerable: "It's hormonal!"

But he still gets nowhere. The moral of the story is that revenge is not so sweet but justice is. And the three wives can best do justice by helping other women.

At what age can a woman be said to be "hormonal"? It's not a simple answer.

Menopause is arbitrarily defined as "the final cessation of menstruation," as if it were a single point in time when the switch is turned off on those fabulous egg-ripening machines, the ovaries. In fact, it's a much more gradual, stop-start series of pauses in ovarian function that are part of that mysterious process called aging.

More changes probably take place during this passage than at any other time in a woman's adult life. It is fortunate, then, that this passage takes some years to complete. As one moves through the physical, psychological, social and spiritual aspects of the transition, dramatic shifts in perspective occur. There may be a transformation in the sense of time, of self in relation to others, and a rethinking of the negative vs. positive aspects of moving into a new and unfamiliar state of being.

The acute period of biological passage, or ovarian transition, spans five to seven years—usually forty-seven or forty-eight to the mid-fifties. But it is the beginning of a long and little-mapped stage of post-reproductive life.

I propose three demarcations of this Second Adulthood for contemporary Western women: *perimenopause* (start of the transition); the *menopause* gateway (completion of the ovarian transition); and a stage I will call *postmenopause and coalescence*—the mirror image of adolescence—in which women can tap into the new vitality Margaret Mead called "postmenopausal zest."

I know what you're thinking. *Thank God this is a book that I don't have to read.* Because you're not fifty yet, or even close. That's the first misconception.

"You're Not Old Enough"

＄

*W*e are born with all the eggs we'll ever have, about seven hundred thousand. Each month after puberty, one ovary offers up a selection of from twenty to one thousand mature eggs, though usually only one is released into the fallopian tube to meet any sperm in the vicinity. As we get close to the bottom of the egg basket, ovulation doesn't always take place. The quality of egg follicles that month may be substandard, or there may not be sufficient estrogen manufactured by the ovaries. When the supply of viable eggs is gone, menstruation stops completely and the fertile period of a woman's life ends.

The median age at which women in Western countries stop ovulating altogether is 50.8. But today there are no clear age cues to when the long transition begins or when it ends. "For a long time we've thought of menopause as a very sudden event—it really isn't," says Dr. Trudy Bush, epidemiologist and associate professor of obstetrics and gynecology at

Johns Hopkins Medical School. "The ovaries start producing less estrogen probably in the mid-thirties. There's a gradual loss of estrogen production and other hormones until the ovaries finally stop putting out very much estrogen at all. It's not uncommon to see symptoms in the early forties as a sign of gradual estrogen withdrawal."

Eight women out of every one hundred undergo a natural menopause *before age forty,* according to renowned reproductive endocrinologist Dr. Lila Nachtigall, director of the Women's Wellness Division at New York University Medical School. The youngest case on record was seen at Kings College Hospital: a nineteen-year-old girl.

Increasingly, say veteran practitioners, the American women turning up in menopause clinics are younger by four or five years than in the recent past. Researchers now admit they have underestimated the number of younger women who experience all the symptoms of menopause even though they still have periods. Some speculate that in the past, when women had many pregnancies, they had an easier menopause. As middle-class Western women we have changed our lifestyle—postponing childbirth, having fewer children, synthetically controlling our menstrual cycle, and often introducing fertility drugs, or having tubes tied or a uterus surgically removed—and we may be throwing our hormonal systems out of balance.

My own younger sister started missing periods when she was forty-three—five years earlier than it began with me. One month her "little friend" would come, then not again for another two or three months, whereupon it would reappear, only to disappear again. After half a year of this, feeling poorly, she called her gynecologist and popped the obvious question: "Is this the beginning of menopause?"

"No," he stated categorically. "You're not old enough."

It's tempting to take this bromide so commonly dispensed by physicians and to go away feeling smug and secure in one's continuing fecundity. Isn't it reassuring to know that you're still young? Well, not *young* exactly, but still, in some respect at least, *underage.*

"I started very early, at forty," I was told by another woman I'll call Barbara, a delightfully wise Oregonian with a thriving psychotherapy practice. "It was no fun. I was blown away by the hot flashes. I felt enormous restlessness, and cranky, cranky, cranky!" Her doctor, too, said she wasn't old enough to take estrogen. Or, as she heard it, she hadn't suffered enough.

A roaring extrovert, Barbara stood up to her full five feet nine inches and stared down her doctor. "Either you give me estrogen, or the next time I have a hot flash I'm going to rip my clothes off and shout your name!"

The man dispensed the pills and preserved his anonymity, but once on hormones, Barbara blew up. "I gained five pounds a year for six years until I finally said the hell with it. I quit taking the estrogen, and I have all the lines in my face to show for it." Now in her early fifties, she does look parched and abruptly elderly. "You age faster after menopause," she concludes, though it would be more accurate to say that one ages faster after any *abrupt* withdrawal from hormones.

On the opposite end, women may never be quite

sure when, or if, they have finished with menopause. This is particularly true for women who go right onto hormone therapy at the first signs of the Change and continue having periods as if they were still reproductive. There is no noticeable evidence of when they stop ovulating, no clear metaphysical marker that they are moving beyond fertility into another stage of life.

Margaret Mead originated the memorable phrase, *postmenopausal zest.* Yet Mary Catherine Bateson, the daughter of the pioneering anthropologist, is still puzzled about when her own mother actually became menopausal. When Dr. Mead reached the age of forty-eight and probably experienced the first hot flashes, she persuaded her doctor to try giving her shots of estrogen, the primary female hormone, telling him it was for a circulatory problem. "And it worked," she noted in a brief medical history made available to me by her daughter, an anthropological researcher and author in her own right. At age fifty-three Dr. Mead noted "longer space between periods and lighter flow." But she continued to have hormone-induced periods for another eight years, whereupon she asserted that she had held off menopause until her sixties.

Most educated women today expect to take control of this annoying little disruption. After all, they have been accustomed to birth control and using technology to correct and control problems with fertility. No wonder so many are thrown into a fit when their bodies unexpectedly backfire on them.

At forty-eight, Lisa Menzies Corletto, a Southern California writer, suddenly found herself in the midst of a maelstrom. She was suffering from depression, sexual discomfort, insomnia. "Every day I would say to myself, 'I'm dying here!'" she admits. "Normal problems had become major life events to be worried about constantly. I had been to psychiatrists, psychologists, gynecologists and my general physician. It seemed there was nothing I could do or take, no one I could see or anything I could learn that would pull me from this quicksand."

Through her own determination to save her mind, her marriage, her life, Corletto continued seeking answers. Finally, as she later wrote to me, she stumbled across *The Silent Passage* and recognized the all-too-familiar symptoms of menopause. "Not in my wildest dreams had I ever imagined menopause could be so devastating, so insidious.

"I immediately made an appointment with my doctor. When he walked into the room I blurted out, 'I think I'm premenopausal and I would like to go on hormone therapy!' He looked at my chart and said, 'You're too young.' I said 'Young? I'm almost fifty!'" Within days of receiving a prescription for HRT, her symptoms were relieved and a semblance of balance and manageability returned to her life.

There is another reason that menopause is no longer clearly linked to middle age today. More than one-third of the women in the United States have hysterectomies—thirty-seven women out of one hundred—an astounding figure. (North America leads the world in numbers of hysterectomies, with twice as many as in Great Britain.) The majority of these women have hysterectomies between the ages of twenty-five and forty-four. A classical hysterectomy, which means removal of the uterus and cervix, *even without removal of the ovaries,* usually brings on an early menopause, within two years of the surgery. Removal of the ovaries, called oophorectomy, brings on menopause immediately, no matter how young a woman is.

This is all part of a fundamental change in the way we view the adult life cycle of women. *The biological transition of menopause is no longer an age-tied marker event.*

But no matter when the first awareness dawns on a woman that menopause might be imminent for *her*, it comes as a shock. Virtually nothing prepares most women for this mysterious and momentous transition. Indeed, some of us unconsciously tell ourselves, "It's not going to happen to me."

When You Least Expect It

❧

*N*o more incongruous time or place could be imagined, the night I was hit by the first bombshell of the battle with menopause. It was a Sunday evening. Snug inside a remarriage not yet a year old, I was sitting utterly still, reading, in a velvet-covered armchair. A pillow's throw away my husband was doing the same, while jazz lapped at our ears and snow curtained the window. Every so often we looked up and congratulated ourselves on staying home in this cocoon of comfort and safeness and love we had created.

Then the little grenade went off in my brain. A flash, a shock, a sudden surge of electrical current that whizzed through my head and left me feeling shaken, nervous, off-balance.

"What was that?" I must have mumbled.

"What?"

"Nothing."

But some powerful switch had been thrown. I tried to go back to reading. It was difficult to concentrate.

When I looked down at the pages I had just finished, I realized the imprint of their content on my brain had washed out. I felt hot, then clammy. I tried lying down, but sleep could not soak up the agitation. My heart was racing, but from what? Complete repose? I felt, for perhaps the first time in my life since the age of thirteen, profoundly ill at ease inside my body.

In the months that followed, I sometimes felt *outside* my body. I was aware of spates of "static" in my brain and came to recognize the aura that preceded the first migraine-like headaches I'd ever had. Usually optimistic, I began having little bouts of blues. Then little crashes of fatigue. Having always counted on abundant energy, it was profoundly upsetting to find myself sometimes crawling home from a day of writing and falling into bed for a "nap," from which I had to drag myself up just to have dinner.

I was only forty-eight. And still menstruating. So this couldn't be the "Change of Life," could it?

Besides, all these strange physical sensations were only background noise in what was otherwise a thrilling, adrenaline-pumping, mind-stretching period of creative redirection, in both my career and my new family life. I was traveling all over the country and the world and coming home to a husband and a new adopted child, both of whom I adored, satisfied that another beloved daughter was already launched into adulthood. So I took Scarlett's "fiddle-dee-dee" approach; I'd think about it tomorrow.

But "tomorrow" I began to notice something strange. For the first time since my early teens, when the sexual pilot light went on and I was warned not to want sex too much, I began to worry about not wanting it enough. Again, I had the sensation of standing outside my body and scolding it: "What's the matter with you—why don't you *act* the way I feel anymore?"

I went to see my conservative, male gynecologist, known as a superb clinician but short on communication skills. He measured my hormone levels. I was very low on estrogen. I vaguely remembered my family doctor having mentioned in passing, when he'd rattled off the results of my annual physical in recent years, that my estrogen levels were getting lower and lower.

"Could I be a candidate for hormone replacement therapy?" I asked.

"Not yet." My gynecologist went strictly by the book. "You're not in menopause, because you're still menstruating. You have to be menstruation-free for a year before I can give you estrogen replacement."

"But this, um, effect on my sexual response"—embarrassed, I fumbled for the words—"couldn't that be because I need more estrogen, like a vitamin supplement?"

"It's nothing I can help you with. Decrease in sexual response is just a natural part of aging."

The curt clinician washed his hands of me. I left his office feeling as though I'd just been handed a one-way ticket to the Dumpster. *Does this mean I can't be me anymore?*

It was time for me to shop for another gynecologist. A recommendation sent me to see Patricia Allen, a vivacious woman and an attending physician at the New York Hospital who demands excellence of herself and discipline from her patients. She made it clear from the start that she does not accept passive patients or women who smoke, only those who are willing to participate actively in their own health care. That sounded reasonable. She spent a good twenty minutes before the physical exam taking a holistic history. The irregular periods, the erratic expanding and constricting of blood vessels that caused the static, and the mood swings indicated to her that I was in perimenopause. Then she said something startling:

"I believe in treating each patient as an individual. This perimenopausal period should be a transformation, so that a woman gets to become—physically, emotionally, and spiritually—the best that she ever was." Imagine your run-of-the-mill male gynecologist harboring such a radical point of view!

Dr. Allen posited that the impact of low estrogen on me, as on many women, was emotional. Of the several hundred patients who consult her about managing their menopause, quite a few mention feeling depressed although they have no rational reason to be. She also took seriously my distress over changes in libido. She asked if there was a history of osteoporosis in my family, which brought to mind memories of my mother suffering in her seventies as she sat on her powdery bones.

All in all, Dr. Allen felt I was a good candidate for hormone therapy, but she drove a strict bargain with her patients. Estrogen by itself carries a known increase in the risk of cancer of the endometrium—the lining of the uterus—which is sloughed during menstrual periods. So she also prescribed a progestin*

---

*The terms are so similar as to be endlessly confusing: Progesterone refers to the natural hormone made by the body to control the action of estrogen; a progestin is any one of the synthetic equivalents; and just to drive you crazy, Europeans call their synthetics progestogens. From here on, I shall use the term progesterone in all cases.

(synthetic progesterone), to protect against that risk. Also, I would have to agree to have an endometrial biopsy several months later to detect any changes in the tissue. She urged me to have a bone density evaluation done ($250), as well as a mammogram. This complete diagnostic workup cost $800, much of which was reimbursable by health insurance. It was costly, but it turned out to be part of an investment in long-term health and productivity that has more than paid for itself—and one I would recommend for all women who can afford it.

I filled the standardized prescription for 0.625 mg of Premarin (estrogen made from pregnant mares' urine, from which it derives its unforgettable name) and 10 mg tablets of Provera, the progesterone that stimulates the sloughing of the uterine lining. This is an approximation of the two hormones that the body produces naturally in the reproductive years.

After only a month, the estrogen had rekindled sexual desire, stopped the surges of static and dips of fatigue, and chased away the blues. But the Provera was another matter. It brought on physical and emotional symptoms that I'd never experienced before. After a year of the combined hormones, my body seemed to be at war with itself for half of every month. My energy was flagging, and resistance to minor infections was falling. I felt as if I were racing my motor. So I stopped taking hormones cold turkey.

Dr. Allen agreed it was a good idea to take a break and see how my body responded. If nothing else, she said, going off hormones often serves to remind women why they started taking them in the first place.

For the first two months off hormones I felt marvelous; the bloating disappeared, as did the induced periods, and the terrible cramps and tension and sleeplessness that had begun to accompany them. I even got my waist back. Then, a crash. All the perimenopausal phenomena returned with exaggerated force. Now the static became full-fledged hot flashes and night sweats that interrupted sleep and left me limp by morning. I went back to my estrogen pills.

Within days the "blue-meanie" moods lifted. I was able to write for twelve hours straight on deadline and remain calm and reasonable under crisis. Within a few weeks all the other complaints were gone. I was staggered by the potency of the female hormone.

But the impact of the progesterone was also intensified. On day fifteen, when I had to add the Provera pills to my regimen, I felt by afternoon as if I had a terrible hangover. This chemically induced state was not to be subdued by aspirin or a walk in the park. It only worsened as the day wore on, bringing with it a racing heart, irritability, waves of sadness, and difficulty concentrating. And to top it off, the hot flashes came back! Cramps introduced pain for a week at a time. By night I couldn't go to sleep without a glass of wine, and even then was awakened by a racing heartbeat and sweating. *Won't I ever be me anymore?*

Taking synthetic progesterone with the estrogen for half of each month was like pushing down the gas pedal and putting on the brakes at the same time, and it left my body confused and worn out.

Clinicians I later interviewed relayed common side effects reported by patients who were taking the drug: "Whenever I take Provera, I have migraines, bloating, breast tenderness, the blues. I feel awful and want to die." More than one woman has said to me, "Why am I going through this for ten days a month? Who needs it?"

Both Dr. Allen and I have learned a great deal since I began my perimenopausal passage. Women and their doctors no longer are limited to the old cyclical regimen I have just described, which still works well for some people. We now have more options. One of the most well-received of these is continuous HRT; that is, instead of going off estrogen for five days at the end of the month and shocking your system by taking big slugs of progesterone, you take the standard dose of estrogen along with a much smaller dose of natural micronized progesterone *every day*. It eventually eliminates periods and maintains a more even balance of hormones—and moods!

The good news is women today don't have to go through the lengthy and painful experimentation that I had to—if they are well-informed. You can now custom-design your own hormone replacement therapy. The Food and Drug Administration (FDA) has approved both options described above. Women are now much more likely to ask for and receive treatment for disruptive symptoms earlier in the lead-up to menopause. In the *Prevention* survey, "We found it especially interesting that so many perimenopausal women (40 percent) had tried hormones," says Dr. Cristina Matera, assistant professor of clinical obstetrics and gynecology at Columbia University. "That's a change in the way physicians approach hormone replacement therapy."

Almost all women experience some menopausal

symptoms, but few have severe problems. An estimated 20 percent sail through with little difficulty and another 10 percent or so are temporarily incapacitated. The rest of us—70 percent of all women— wrestle to some degree with difficulties that come and go over a period of years as we deal with the long transition from our reproductive state. (Data going back to the nineteenth century are consistent: Almost all women experience some menopausal symptoms, but few have severe problems.)

Hormone replacement therapy is currently taken by 20 to 25 percent of American women age forty-five and over who are menopausal, a significant increase over the last several years. In 1997, over forty-five million prescriptions were written for Premarin. More than 14.2 million were dispensed for Prempro, a combination of Premarin and progesterone.

To come up with a safe and intelligent custom design for your menopause, however, means you will have to do most of the work (see section on Hormone Replacement Therapy in "Should I or Shouldn't I?"). Find a doctor who is making a special effort to keep abreast of developments in this rapidly changing area of medicine. Many women, however, are woefully ignorant about the intelligent questions to ask a doctor. What is right for you today might have serious conscquences five years from now, so even after you do some research or experimentation and find the solution for you, it is still important to keep up to date on the research findings coming out.

Cinderella Hits Menopause

❧

*A*s the pacesetters among baby boom generation women discover menopause on their horizon, they are bringing it out of the closet. One of the earliest group discussions took place in Los Angeles in 1991—a conversation that in a previous generation would have been unimaginable.

It seems that my article had stirred up a little *frisson* of fright among some of the movers and shakers in the film community. In that world, where leading ladies never look a day over twenty-nine and studio executives start subtracting years from their résumés before they hit thirty, Hollywood producer Lynda Guber had picked up a copy of *Vanity Fair* and discovered a cloud on the horizon of her perfect existence.

"Menopause!" she shrieked. "God, I've never seen that word written."

Lynda is a sizzling redhead from Brooklyn who reached the pinnacle of Hollywood society together with her husband, Peter Guber, producer of *Batman* and *Rainman,* former head of SONY Pictures Entertainment and now head of his own production company. The next day she bumped into Joanna Poitier at a Beverly Hills bistro and asked innocently, "How are you doing?"

"I'm a lunatic, I'm going through menopause and empty nest at the same time," said the beautiful actress-wife of actor Sidney Poitier. (It is culture-specific in Hollywood to identify women by their husbands' professional status.)

This is fantastic, thought Lynda. *This woman is ready to talk about how she feels.* Lynda herself had already decided "the impact of menopause will not be devastating on me, that's what my holistic belief system tells me," but all she knew about it, in fact, was that the subject was a real no-no. Lynda is committed to being a consciousness-raiser of people in the movie business, having cofounded an organization, Education 1st!, that spreads positive messages through TV shows. She passed the word to a friend, Annie Gilbar, then editor of *LA Style.* "Annie, I have an idea. I'd like to have a meeting on menopause with the girls." The first invitees backed off. Word spread, and before long it became such a cachet event there had to be a luncheon and a dinner group. I was invited to come out and speak to both. My friend and gynecologist, Dr. Patricia Allen, accompanied me.

Going to Hollywood to talk about menopause was a little bit like going to Las Vegas to sell savings accounts. Such is the obsession with youthfulness in Southern California, one half expects there to be an ordinance against menopause there. "Women who are menopausal in California are around the bend—they view it like cancer," I was warned by a Chinese medicine specialist with a deluxe and desperate clientele in Los Angeles.

Nevertheless, it was a golden opportunity. California women in the boomer vanguard are normally the most uninhibited among their species in speaking out about whatever bothers them. I quickly discovered, however, that even they—women who have access to the most up-to-date information, women who are religious about doing the stations of their Nautilus machines, women who have phone indexes of dozens of doctors, not to mention the best acupuncturists, herbalists, liposuctionists, and shrinks—*even they* didn't have any answers on menopause. In fact, they had never discussed the questions, even among themselves. When they did come together to confront the subject, they reflected many of the secret fears and defensive reactions common among women everywhere.

Lynda invited us to gather at her Japanese-style fantasy beach house. At the door each woman was invited to leave her shoes on a shelf and choose a kimono. I kept looking for a gray hair in the crowd— scarcely a one among this mostly blond, mid-fortyish group. The guests draped themselves over big black cushions on tansu boxes in the screening room. It was reminiscent of slumber parties in junior high school, when girls played dress-up and talked about taboo subjects like sex. But now we were grownups; and the very fact these prominent women had showed up, in this subculture, was an act of bravery.

"I invited Glenn Close to come," said one of the women. "I thought she was going to faint dead away."

I began by asking those present to introduce themselves, give their age, and say why they had come—what meaning did menopause have for them? The wife of one of the town's top studio executives confessed she usually shunned "negative subjects," but her mother was dead and she had no one else to consult. A woman who heads her own company described herself as an information junkie. "My gynecologist tells me that I'm not going through the Change at all, but I know my body, and I feel different over the past year. I've had occasional night sweats. I used to think I had a virus."

Lisa Specht, a lawyer, has no children and said she didn't think she had to worry about menopause, at least until she was fifty-five or something. "I haven't had any symptoms yet, except that my skin has been oily," she assured herself.

The outspoken Joanna Poitier broke the ice. She was willing to admit she might be going through menopause, although her primary concern was letting go of her two daughters, now eighteen and twenty. "I keep waking up in the middle of the night, changing my nightgown. I went to the gynecologist, and she told me that I was still moist. She said I won't probably go into menopause for another two years. I have night sweats. I tried it without the duvet and the nightgown, and I still have night sweats. I have day sweats, too! The back of my neck is damp all day long."

The next speaker was immediately recognizable. Lesley Ann Warren, the movie actress we all remember from her ethereal portrayal of Cinderella in the TV musical, is even more beautiful today. Her features are still delicate, her body is still slim and supple, and reddish brown hair ripples over her shoulders. More appealing than all that are the quickened intelligence and candor that she has earned over forty years and brought to her more recent roles in the films *Victor/Victoria,* and *Choose Me.* But Lesley Ann makes her living here in Cinderella Land, where girls are never supposed to grow up. Hollywood ruthlessly cuts the finest actresses once they reach forty—yes, even Meryl! Studio executives will callously describe a thirty-eight-year-old actress who is still gorgeous as "over the hill" or "She's an old hag." As an actress in that workplace, Lesley Ann Warren is torn between her liberated feminist beliefs and the devastating reality that every day her worth is judged by her age and her looks.

Divorced from Jon Peters, former cohead of the former Columbia Studios, with whom she had a son, Lesley Ann had been single for some time. She now had a new love. It was he who found a photocopy of my *Vanity Fair* article lying around. Lesley Ann wanted to educate herself on the subject before it happened so she could deal with it homeopathically and herbally, as she does everything else. She had forgotten to hide the evidence.

"You know, I read this article," he said casually one night.

Ohmigod, he's found me out! was the actress's first thought. "I was really scared he would think *I* was menopausal. I felt ashamed." But he surprised her.

"I'm glad I read it. I feel like any man who's in a relationship with a woman dealing with this must be very loving, very aware, and very present," he said.

Lesley Ann counted her new love among an ultramicroscopic subspecies of the male genus, at least as they are bred by the movie business. "In all the rest of my experience, men are so staggeringly uneducated in this area, it's deadly for us," she told the group. "Most men I know run from the word *menopause.*"

"We're afraid to educate the men, that's our problem," amended Joanna. "I have never been afraid to say how old I am. I've never had surgery or collagen or anything like that. And I don't feel any less terrific because I'm menopausal. Whoever you are with, they should experience the whole thing that you're experiencing." Joanna added vociferously, "I take no aspirin, no Tylenol; if I have a headache, I live through it. I don't believe in pills. I know that I will not take hormones, because to me it's unnatural."

The word *holistic* was almost a fetish in this group. Used indiscriminately, it might mean one who never uses Tylenol, or one who has stopped taking drugs and alcohol, or one who consults Chinese medical doctors and herbalists but *never* a member of the American Medical Association. A bouncy talent agent with a blond boy-cut admitted she was taking hormones; *admitted,* because, like so many women, her decision was tinged with guilt. "I knew something was up when I went to a restaurant and had to ask the waiter for two menus—one to see what I was ordering and the other to fan myself."

Knowing laughter rippled through the group. We decided that if we met again we would call ourselves The Fan Club.

The agent revealed a more intimate reason for her decision. "One night when my husband and I were having sex, it felt like I was a virgin. I said, 'Something is wrong here.' My gynecologist took a blood test and told me it was the Change of Life." She emphasized that she was on a very low dose of hormone replacement therapy and that she was happy with the results.

Joanna Poitier broke in with a question on everybody's mind. "Is it okay to go through the rest of life without estrogen?"

Dr. Allen said there was no definitive answer. "When we are in this part of our lives, we have to make decisions about what it is that we want. Beyond the symptomatic discomforts, there are also medical issues that bear on our long-term health—osteoporosis, heart disease, breast and uterine cancer." Dr. Allen's advice was to gather as much information as possible, including that concerning one's own family history, to find out if there is a medical reason to take hormone replacement therapy, and then make a decision.

"But we don't have to make a decision for life. We make a decision for three months, and then we make a decision again," she added, sowing visible relief in some of the tense faces. Others were impatient with this answer. They had come looking for a risk-free, all-natural curative.

Mary Miccuci introduced herself as a "stress queen." A tall, Cher-like streak of a woman who started her own catering business, Along Came Mary, she dashes around Hollywood putting on spreads for the stars. Her signs of menopause began with palpitations; she thought she was having a heart attack. "The quality of my life is changing—all of our lives are changing. I want information!" she said angrily, pitching forward to lean her elbows on her knees. "I want to go through this process as quickly as possible. I'm on a holistic journey to deal with it. Are there the right herbs to take care of the silent killers—heart disease and osteoporosis?"

Surely what they all wanted to hear from me and Dr. Allen was that some magic regimen—yoga and yogurt, or yams and ginseng and green leafy vegetables—would allow them to remain exactly as they had been: youthful wives, sexually appealing and responsive lovers, efficient career builders. They were not yet ready to consider a new self-definition. And until one is ready to do so, the information that is available is not much use.

"I think that we have all been too passive about what the outcome of our lives should be," Mary continued huffily. "Because I tell you, the way I felt for a year was pretty shitty. I have a five-and-a-half-year-old little girl, and I want to be so together for this kid. This menopause stuff, I'll be goddamned if I'll let it get in my way."

Mary's hostility toward the whole subject was revelatory. She had become used to managing her life like a man, according to goals, timetables, balance sheets. She was a businesswoman accustomed to efficiency; in fact, she had to leave early to cater a screening party for Bette Midler's latest film. But now, at the peak of her productivity, she was feeling violated by this reassertion of her body's biologic identity. There is nothing efficient about "this menopause stuff."

Aloma Ichinose, a photographer equally active in her career, had taken the opposite approach. "I'm going through the Change right now. I feel great about it. But at first it was a nightmare. I was raised by a man so none of this was ever talked about." Allowing time for trial and error, Aloma had made several different decisions over the previous year. When urine and blood tests confirmed that she was in menopause, her doctor put her on Premarin. To her, it felt like doing drugs. "I did the Premarin for six months. I felt wonderful, and all my symptoms—the disrupted sleep, the forgetfulness—went away." She added defensively, "I'm not into drugs. I haven't had a drink in years. But I was really worried about bone loss. I'm active, I'm a photographer, I need my strength." Eventually the fear and guilt over taking hormones got to her, and after the six months she stopped. "And all the symptoms returned," she admitted. "I just didn't feel well, and so I'm back on it again and I feel good."

An art gallery owner pressed the issue of age prevention. "How long do you take this? Will it prolong our youth? We are young in our forties, where people of other generations weren't. I'm forty-seven years old, but I don't think that I am forty-seven in numbers. I have the same energy as always."

Joanna, whose blond tendrils and soft curves help her to maintain the jolly all-American-girl good looks of a perpetual cheerleader, is able to maintain the illusion of her inner eye: "I still feel like I'm twenty-eight. I wear my hair the same way, I'm twenty-eight years old."

Another woman in the room muttered, "But you're not. And they *know* you're not."

It cut like a flesh wound into the self-image of every woman there. They were all attractive, and that statement didn't even need the qualifying prefix *still*. External beauty wasn't the real problem. It was the dysynchrony between their idealized inner images— the women they were at their nubile peaks—and blanks where the faces and bodies and spirits of their future selves would have to be filled in, sooner or later. As vanguard baby boomers they agreed, they belonged to the most pampered, narcissistic, and obstinately adolescent generation in American history. "We have delayed duty, responsibility, and commitment," wrote a spokeswomen for their generation, Lynn Smith, in the *Los Angeles Times*. "We have dieted, jogged, and exercised so much, we look and actually *think* we are five to ten years younger than we are."

The most telling reaction of all came from a sleek-looking South African woman who had been mute all night. Before I left, she took me aside and asked the quintessential Southern California question:

"Tell me, what can I do so I *don't have to have this?*"

It was agreed that the vestigial attitude surrounding menopause—"I'm no good anymore"—would be changed by the way women like themselves handled it. I suggested, only half seriously, "If every woman in menopause told five people in the next week, those five people would have an entirely different view of it. 'This dish is in menopause? Well, maybe it isn't so terrible.'" Dr. Allen observed that at this stage we have responsibilities to the world, not just to our tiny communities. She is excited every day by finding new channels to educate women about their bodies. "That's my public passion," she said. "But we also need something for ourselves—new passions all the time."

I added wickedly, "And they may include a twenty-five-year-old lover."

"Yeah, a *blind* twenty-five-year-old lover!" amended one of the California women.

With a whooping and shimmying of laughter, the session ended. Seventeen women went out into the world to resume their balancing acts among careers, husbands, children, car pools, social and spiritual lives, too busy to worry much about menopause, but better prepared for the future. Laughter and forgetting . . . two of the best gifts women of any age can share with one another.

But something hopeful, something even incendiary had come out of this session with California women. Their need to know was beginning to overcome their fear of knowing.

Deal or Deny?

∽

"When I turned fifty, I cried a lot," said a New York businesswoman. "You have to grieve, and then when you come out on the other side, it feels very liberating."

Singer-songwriter Joni Mitchell described to me the pits-to-peak course of her passage in much the same way. "I went over the hump of the middle-life crazies. There is a kind of mourning period for those things you can no longer do. But then something happened of its own accord. You can feel a chemical change in your body, as you go over that hump. You have a greater ability to let go and say, 'I don't want to think about that now,' which is the thing I always admired about men."

Psychologist Ellen McGrath, a vivacious and experienced media spokeswoman in her mid forties and a good friend of mine, was preparing to go out on her first book tour. She was petrified. She had drawn for three years on all her physical and mental resources to produce her magnum opus on depression, a book for the popular market titled *When Feeling Bad Is Good.* Now she had to go out and sell it; no tryouts out of town, she had to open on a national breakfast TV show before an audience of five million.

"The week before the tour, suddenly I couldn't remember my material. Pieces of it would just go. I thought, 'My God, my mind is the main thing I have. What's happening to me?'"

Ellen had recently been having trouble sleeping, feeling vaguely hot but without sweating. Earlier, I had shared with her some of my research. "Though I never thought it would apply to me," she later confessed, "I did have some hunch of what this could be, and a name for my malaise—menopause." So she asked her doctor to fit her in immediately and had a blood test done to measure her hormone levels. "Turns out, I wasn't just in *peri*menopause. I had gone straight into full menopause, at forty-six!" The doctor gave her an injection of a megadose of estrogen to hold her over for several months. "The astounding thing was, my symptoms disappeared within forty-eight hours," says Ellen.

But after this quick fix, those symptoms reappeared with a vengeance. Ellen was enraged. "I don't have time to deal with this!" she insisted. Having recently been there myself, I knew exactly how she felt: she was losing some of the control she'd fought so hard to gain. It's particularly dispiriting to feel a loss of control over something so elemental as our bodies.

"You can't run away from it," I tried to tell Ellen. "What you have to do at this stage is go home. Listen to your body. Take the pause—you've earned it."

But my friend couldn't buy my argument. Not then, at any rate. She was angry—who isn't at first? But her response was not to deal with it but to deny it. "I don't have time for menopause!" she screamed. "I just want postmenopause zest."

These are normal, predictable reactions to the first phase of menopause, especially for the achieving women of the Baby Boom. You will be angry, embarrassed, impatient, and incredulous that this could happen to you. You may believe that if you do give in to menopause, your identity will disintegrate, along with your body, and you will turn into a dried-up old crone overnight.

You are not alone. Hundreds of women I have interviewed felt the same way at the outset of this passage. The late forties often represent the pits for women, while the early fifties usually find them at their peak. Before one breaks into that most productive stage of life, one must accept losses of certain powers taken for granted in earlier stages. The youthful looks you could always trade on, and the magical powers of procreation that connected you to the cycle of all life—these are the God-given, gloriously unfair advantages of being born a well-formed woman. Suddenly, in the mid-forties, one must face the fact that these powers are ebbing.

"For many of us who waited until we were well into our thirties and even early forties before having children, the physical power of giving birth is still palpable; it touches something very deep and instinctual," ventured Suzanne Rosenblatt Buhai, a Los Angeles psychotherapist. "That flame of the instinctual being extinguished is not as readily dealt with as one might think."

Dealing with loss is one of the tasks we struggle with in every passage, but it is particularly poignant as women notice the first skips in a fertility we have probably taken for granted. The feelings were brought out by a woman who has obviously delighted in maternity. Joyce Bogart Trabulus has two children and a quartet of stepchildren in her life, and is further fulfilled by community caretaking, running charities for cancer and AIDS research. She has no desire to have any more children. No *daylight world* desire.

"And yet I really feel sadness every time I think about it," she admitted. "I was forty-one when I had my last child, who's three years old now. Sometimes I catch myself thinking, *Oh God, this is fabulous, I'd love to do this again.* It's a great loss to know that it will be impossible for me. It's not like I want another one. And I'm not menopausal, or even premenopausal. But I look at a baby and say, 'Oh.'"

Dr. Buhai mused out loud, "Given our generational narcissism—whether it's because of our sheer numbers, Dr. Spock, or the dominant influence of psychoanalysis—I just wonder if this concern with self is now being focused on menopause. Are we getting all worked up over something that is, in fact, quite normal and has been experienced since time immemorial? Perhaps, the best gift we can give society at this stage is to see this as something very positive. If we can normalize this experience, as Gail says, it will help women deal with it. Otherwise, women will take on the responsibility of this somehow being their fault—they are supposed to be pulling out of this funk."

"Menopause is not a disease," says the epidemiologist Trudy Bush. "It's a life transition, but it carries with it a different internal hormonal milieu which is, in fact, detrimental to our bodies. When we don't have estrogen, our bones get brittle, our rates of heart disease go up, our vagina becomes less moist, our skin becomes dry and thin. In fact, we can reverse those processes that are related to the hormones rather than to aging per se."

Estrogen is involved in something like three hundred bodily processes. So, when it dips below levels one's body has come to rely upon as normal for thirty years or more, the body is naturally thrown out of balance. The brain's brain, the hypothalamus, cannot coordinate with its usual precision functions like body temperature, metabolic rate, sleep cycle, blood chemistry, and so on.

Subtle influences on brain chemistry, similar to the experience of jet lag, may be a harbinger of perimenopause, for instance. The editor of the London *Sunday Express,* Eve Pollard, admits that she sometimes has a little more difficulty concentrating or remembering things these days. "I know I have to make lists, but then I'm running a magazine and a newspaper and trying to manage children and stepchildren as they get older, when you can't lay down the law anymore." In her second marriage, juggling two children and three stepchildren, Pollard may be in for a pleasant surprise.

All but about 10 percent of women, which represents the extreme, will function quite effectively throughout menopause at balancing their usual nine lives. But they must take the trouble to inform themselves, since no one else will. "All of us are quite ignorant," Pollard admits.

The temptation, of course, is to deny the signs. Or to give up on dealing with the larger passage because we can't find quick and easy answers to resolve the physical challenge of menopause. In talking to women all over the United States and Britain, I did find some significant differences in attitudes and reactions to menopause, depending on how women are valued in a particular subculture. But there was one strong common denominator: Most women in midlife are still afraid to know—and fiercely resist acknowledging—that menopause can affect *them,* but at the same time, in spite of themselves, they are desperately anxious to learn what it's all about.

Privately, women will go to extraordinary lengths to pick up information—cornering a researcher at a party and interrogating him, stealing books from doctors' offices—I was particularly proud to learn that *The Silent Passage* made the list of Ten Most Shoplifted Books in America—but heaven forbid that anyone should bring up the subject at the dinner table! Psychologist Abraham Maslow gave a name to this syndrome of ambivalence: "the need to know and the fear of knowing."

In fact, there is no single, risk-free solution that suits everyone. Menopause is highly idiosyncratic. Remember how different we were, one from another, as we entered puberty—some of us embarrassed still to be wearing undershirts at thirteen, while our best friend was turning into a hunchback to hide the pods suddenly swelling under her sweater? Well, the Change of Life is even more individual. Peggy Sue may tell you that she hardly noticed a thing. Her periods tapered off, she had a few hot flashes, but she sailed right through—no problem. Peggy Sue may be one of the lucky 10 or 15 percent of women who find the Change of Life uneventful. She may also be plump, or obese, and since estrogen is produced in the fat cells, this is one case where fat is more advantageous than thin. Or, she may be lying.

Whatever Peggy Sue's experience of the Change, it

doesn't make *your* signs and symptoms any less true. The older we grow, the more *un*like we are from each other. Besides the changes in our brains and sexual characteristics over the years, our endocrine systems are different, our metabolisms are different, our blood vessels and bones become more dissimilar, depending on our lifetime eating and exercise habits. So it is not surprising that there is not *one* menopause; there are hundreds of variations.

But instead of giving in to frustration over dealing with our uniqueness, we can recognize how lucky we are. In all of human history women's lives were under the coercion of their biology. Today we don't have to be forty-five years old and suddenly estrogen-deficient, miserable, and without recourse. We have choices. And they don't all involve taking drugs, by any means.

The first step we can take toward mastering this stage of life is to describe the beast, give a shape and characteristics to it, and look it in the face. The actual derivation of the word menopause is from the Greek *meno,* meaning "month," and *pausis,* which is literally translated "ending," though more accurately it connotes a pause in the life cycle. The Change of Life is one of the three great "blood mysteries" that demarcate a woman's inner life, the earlier ones being menarche and pregnancy.

Despite the trial-and-error state of medical care, a woman at fifty now has a second chance. To use it, she must make an alliance with her body and negotiate with her vanity. Today's healthy, active pacesetters will become the pioneers, mapping out a whole new territory for potent living and wisdom-sharing from one's fifties to one's eighties and even beyond.

Mother Doesn't Always Know Best

❧

"*I* don't know how to be fifty," one West Coast woman told me. "I'm not going to be fifty like my mother, and there haven't really been any models."

Very rarely do any of the women I interview learn much about menopause from their own mothers. If they reported any mother-daughter conversation on the subject at all, the mothers' answers tended to be brief and evasive: "There was nothing to it; my periods just stopped."; or, "I don't remember much about menopause."

Even women in their twenties confide that the subject of menopause is usually discussed at home with ominous overtones. Rebecca Donner, a twenty-six-year-old writer in New York, says, "I grew up hearing about this dark, baleful cloud that descended on my great-grandmother and grandmother in mid-life." But when her mother began to experience menopausal symptoms such as irregular bleeding, the subject was avoided. "She kept going to the doctor for these extensive tests that were always inconclusive, and for a while I was terrified that she was suffering from some horrible, obscure illness. Even though we were having thermostat wars and she was having trouble sleeping, I never quite made the connection that she was going through menopause."

On reflection, Rebecca wondered if her mother felt confronted with an imminent loss. "Given our family's folklore, I don't know whether she was expecting an ax to fall, but since then she has said to me, 'Menopause is something that takes place over a span of time.' She's much more at ease now."

"When I asked my mother about menopause," said Effie Graham, a black nurse who grew up in the South, "all she said was, 'You'll find out when you get it.' She never told me about my period either."

Not surprising. It was common in their day for women in the Change to be institutionalized. "Nervous breakdown" they called it. Because nobody associated their intense depression with menopause and the *temporary* breakdown of hormonal balance.

There are good reasons that the same mothers and mothers-in-law who assume possession of the revealed wisdom on child rearing are peculiarly scanty of expertise on this subject. The mothers of today's menopause-aged women were an exceptionally prudish lot. It was shameful to discuss any bodily functions in their day.

And what was there to discuss about menopause? Our mothers had no information. No biomedical research had been done into the most pressing health questions of women as they age. Most of our mothers had no idea of the major killer diseases or disorders that could deprive them of a decent quality of life in their sixties, seventies, or eighties. And they certainly didn't know that their risk of being attacked by heart disease, hip fractures, and breast cancer was decidedly affected by the way they handled their Change of Life.

It is safe to assume most of our mothers never even heard the word *osteoporosis*—a silent disease caused by deterioration of the bone tissue—much less associated it with menopause. Only in the last five years or so has osteoporosis been identified as a crippler of life's quality, afflicting almost twenty-five million women. It leeches the very lining of our bones, like a colony of termites inside our foundations. Beginning their invisible destruction as soon as our supply of estrogen is depleted, these "termites" accelerate their robbing of minerals from our bones during the time around menopause.

Many women in their forties today are at the hub of several generations. Unless they're incapacitated, they feel too stretched for time and money to consult doctors or take expensive tests in order to manage their own menopause. In fact, most middle-class and low-income women don't consult any professional about how to protect their health and well-being during the Change of Life. If they adopt their mothers' attitudes without examination, they often blindly follow a path that, unbeknownst to the older women, may have been responsible for untold deficits of mental and physical well-being.

Even women whose mothers experienced no apparent problems during menopause may be at some risk if not greater risk than those who are prepared for the worst. If a woman tells her daughter that she will sail through the Change just like she did, the daughter might not take the time to seek proper medical care and prevention.

A forty-four-year-old New York editor describes this dilemma. "My mother took me out to dinner one day about fourteen years ago and said 'I just want you to know, I've gone through menopause and it was very simple. I had a few hot flashes, and I'm not on hormones, and I feel just great.' Do I believe her? I don't know. But both my grandmothers died of heart disease so I know it's an issue for me."

Monkeying
with Evolution

✍

*A*nother reason for the mystery surrounding menopause is that human females today are monkeying with evolution. Most higher primates do not live long enough in the wild even to have a menopause; the phenomenon has never been clearly established in apes or monkeys, according to Kim Wallen, a researcher at Emory University's Yerkes Primate Center. Most female animals just go right on breeding until they roll over and die.

The same was true of human females for many thousands of years. At the turn of the century a woman could expect to live to the age of forty-seven or -eight. She bore an average of eight children, which kept her busy giving birth or nursing right up to the day she died.

Nature, then, never provided for women who would *routinely* live several decades beyond the age of fifty. Once females had made their genetic contribution, evolution was finished with them, and society followed suit. In view of this historically powerful linkage of menopause with decline and death, is it any wonder that today's women approach fifty under a shadow of archetypal fears of being transformed, all at once, into Old Woman?

The secrecy, shame and ignorance that still veil this natural transition have carried over from the Victorian age with very little mitigation of the punishing stereotypes. "Menopause in the nineteenth century was described only in terms of what women lose at this stage of life," says Marilyn Yalom, senior scholar at the Stanford University Institute for Research on Women and Gender. The Victorians were obsessed with women as reproductive creatures. Once barren and widowed, as they were likely to be by fifty, they were cued to view menopause as "the gateway to old age through which a woman passed at the peril of her life." Yalom's chapter in the documentary text *Victorian Women* quotes nineteenth-century obstetricians who taught that "the change of life unhinges the female nervous system and deprives women of their personal charm."

The most famed women writers over the past hundred years have largely ignored, or been ignorant of, menopause. The romantic novels of George Sand, one of the most staggeringly prolific writers of the nineteenth century in the French language, were read as widely as Balzac's and Hugo's throughout the European continent. Sand also penned twenty-five volumes of letters while inspiring the music of her younger lover, Frederic Chopin. Yet in this vast landscape of words scholar Marilyn Yalom has uncovered only two personal letters in which Sand refers to the symptoms of menopause. In the first, written to her editor, Hetzel, in 1853, Sand was forty-nine years old:

> *I am as well as I can be, given the crisis of my age. So far everything has taken place without grave consequence, but with sweats that I find overwhelming, and which are laughable because they are imaginary. I experience the phenomenon of believing that I am sweating 15 or 20 times a day and night . . . I have both the heat and the fatigue. I wipe my face with a white handkerchief and it is laughable because I am not sweating at all. However, that makes me very tired.*

Sand was chiding herself out of ignorance for having hot flashes and night sweats. Often a woman does not perspire, even though she is experiencing an abrupt leap in skin temperature of one or two degrees. "Even today it's very difficult to explain to a woman that it's a real neurophysiological event, not a psychological event at all, and therefore nothing she should be ashamed of," says Dr. Robert Lindsay, an endocrinologist and leading researcher in the field of menopausal medicine at the Helen Hayes Bone Center in West Haverstraw, New York. Not until the mid-1970s were laboratory tests developed that could demonstrate objectively the neurological discharge in the brain that causes the subjective changes women describe. When a woman says, "I am now having a hot flash," a machine similar to an EKG will show a spike in the ink line running across it.

George Sand refused to allow this inconvenience to interrupt her productivity and finished her letter by saying, "Nonetheless I am working and I've just done a play in three acts . . ." Weeks later she indicated in a letter to her son that she had "rounded the horn" and felt better than she had for a long time. Sand was smart enough to know that even she should make a healthy adaptation in the exhausting nocturnal work habits she had devised, as a young mother, to work around domestic duties. "I sleep well, I eat well, I no longer have those flashes and I'm working without fatigue. It is true that I don't give myself to excess anymore and at one o'clock in the morning I wrap myself in my bed without hesitation."

One in the morning, for George Sand, was early. After fifty she stopped writing from midnight to four A.M. But by then she was a polished professional with twenty years of writing behind her, and she was able to ensconce herself at her country estate and produce the many novels for which she is famous. George Sand was still vibrant, and still writing, when she died at the age of seventy-two.

Anaïs Nin, another fearless watchwoman over the back alleys of the female psyche, neglected the subject in her writings. Virginia Woolf's fragile nature was bedeviled by physical illness and mental anguish at every stage. She attracted particularly harsh criticism for the book that expressed her viewpoint as a woman in her fifties, *Three Guineas.* Woolf attributed none of her ills to menopause and never mentioned it in her writings, though she must have passed through it before she took her own life at fifty-nine. Colette was one of the rare writers to mention menopause at all in her work, portraying it in her novel *Break of Day* as both daunting and potentially empowering.

Fast-forward a hundred years and we find the same

kind of fear and shame around hormonal changes—
on the part of men! At least two recent American
presidents have been on hormone replacement therapy. John Kennedy's adrenal glands were almost completely deteriorated. (Without the regulatory hormones the adrenals produce, wasting and death is the
end result.) Even as he campaigned in the watershed
1960 election against Richard Nixon, Kennedy's hormonal condition was kept under control by replacement hormones. A wall of denial and cover stories
kept his adrenal insufficiency and HRT regimen secret
for many years, the silence being broken only in 1992
by two pathologists who conducted the autopsy on
President Kennedy.

Similarly, the public didn't know that George Bush
had started hormone replacement therapy while he
was president. He began acting jittery in the summer
of 1991. The public puzzled over the manic energy he
displayed, racing around in his cigarette boat and
jumping from one sport to another, all the while he
was calling together a worldwide military response to
Saddam Hussein's invasion of Kuwait. The White
House doctor eventually disclosed that the president's
overactive thyroid gland had been treated with radio-
active iodine and destroyed in April 1991 and that he
must take a daily dose of the hormone that his body
no longer makes naturally.

The thyroid hormone is a major regulator of the
body's metabolism. Its functions can be easily maintained by taking the hormone, but the body is highly
sensitive to dosages, and chronic stress or heavy travel
with changing of time zones can throw everything off.
Thus, when Bush began behaving erratically and
making constant verbal gaffes in his speeches at the

height of his summer 1992 reelection campaign, a wave of rumors about his health flooded the stock market. The crisis prompted his doctor, Burton Lee, to disclose to the press that he had recently been "messing around" with Bush's dosage of hormone replacement.

So, even *male* world leaders can have volatile hormones.

Whose Menopause
Is It Anyway?

❦

$\mathcal{I}$s biology destiny? Of course not. But there are militant feminists who want us to believe that, beneath the learned male and female roles that culture lays upon us, all people are essentially similar. Understandably, there is strong resistance to believing that our behavior is influenced by the biochemical balance in our bodies, because it suggests that we have very little free will. It's unfortunate, and silly, to make it an either/or argument. If you ask me, do I believe in free will? I would borrow the answer given by Isaac Bashevis Singer: "Of course, I have no choice."

Animal studies have shown how fickle behavior can be, depending upon the amount of male or female hormone present in either sex. Strong evidence already exists connecting the aggressive behavior of males with the male hormone, testosterone. The more startling observations come from very recent studies of hyenas at the University of California, Berkeley. With other animals, male babies engage in more rough play than females, due to the early testosterone they had circulating during fetal life. In a unique situation in all of biology, the hormonal bath in which female hyena fetuses grow is loaded with estrogen *and* testosterone, as well as androstenedione, a precursor able to be transformed into more fiery doses of testosterone. The females develop a huge clitoris at birth and eventually display a hanging genital that has erections and is indistinguishable from a male penis.

At the hyena pen in Berkeley, I watched the amazing gender-bending behavior that results from this biological switch. No sooner were they born than two females began tearing each other apart. When the third female of triplets emerged, she was barely an hour old before her sisters began chewing at her birth sac. The point was observable before our very eyes: high testosterone accounts for aggressive behavior in both males and females.

As they age, the female hyenas' level of testosterone dips well below that of the males'. Notwithstanding, the females continue to be the more pugnacious and to remain in charge of their animal hierarchy. Dr. Lawrence Frank and Dr. Steven Glickman, animal behaviorists coordinating the study, tossed a huge hunk of horse meat into the pen of the young adults. The ranking female leapt on it and began reducing it to a grease spot, while the male laid back, passively, until she'd had her fill. "At this point, he defers to her without giving it a second thought," observed Dr. Glickman. By then, learned behavior has taken over from hormones. Thus does it remain difficult to disentangle culture from hormonal effects.

A clear link has been established, for example, between estrogen and women's verbal superiority, just as there is a link between testosterone and men's facility with math and visual-spatial tasks. The levels of hormone matter as well. When women of reproductive age were studied recently, their verbal dexterity was found to peak in the middle of their monthly cycle—just when estrogen levels were at their highest. Immediately after they finished menstruating, when circulating estrogen was at its lowest monthly ebb, their speed on verbal tasks declined. Even at their lowest speed, however, most of the women outperformed men on all verbal tests. By the same token, pubescent boys who have abnormally low levels of testosterone do poorly on spatial tasks.

In pulling together these recent studies, anthropologist Helen E. Fisher, author of *Anatomy of Love: The Natural History of Monogamy, Adultery, and Divorce*, proposes that these subtle gender differences make evolutionary sense. When ancestral males squatted in the African veldt to watch and hunt animals many millennia ago, those who were best in the visual-spatial skills of mapping and tracking might well have survived disproportionately. Similarly, ancestral women needed minute manual dexterity to pick seeds and berries out of the dense vegetation, while verbal skills may have been critical to communicating with their young; again, selecting for these traits in modern women.

"For decades, if not centuries, scientists in search of an understanding of human nature have used male behavior as a benchmark and compared all data on females with this standard," writes Fisher, pointing out this is why we have known almost nothing about the biological tendencies of women. Now that we are just beginning to learn, it would be a shame to throw out the baby with the ancestral bathwater. Fisher makes a good case from anthropological findings that the two sexes survived by teaming up and sharing one another's biological advantages. ". . . our ancestors had begun to collect, butcher, and share meat. The sexes had started to make their living as a team . . . this hunting-gathering lifestyle would produce an intricate balance between women, men and power."

Is There a
Male Menopause?

☙

𝒯he question inevitably comes up, is there a male menopause? Yes, but there are important differences. All men do not become infertile at around the same age, and some men continue to have sufficient testosterone to sire children well into older age. Nevertheless, according to leading endocrinologists I have consulted, a decline in sexual prowess is a clear phenomenon among men, and it is correlated with a decline in testosterone levels. Dr. Pentti Siiteri, former professor and codirector of the Reproductive Endocrinology Center at the University of California, San Francisco, and an authority on hormonal mechanisms, explains, "This is analogous to what happens to a female, the significant difference being there is no sharp demarcation point; therefore, it is impossible to define when the decline in sexual prowess starts. Most men," he adds, "begin to taper off in their mid-fifties to sixties."

But they don't talk about it. Not to their wives. Not

even to other men. "Because you don't want to admit weakening," adds Dr. Lawrence Frank. "Your job as a male is to be strong."

"Sooner or later, however, virtually *all* men will have a male menopause," states Dr. Siiteri. "It's the difference between a gradual decline and a more abrupt one."

Now here's the good news for women. Biology at the Change of Life works to women's advantage. The turmoil wrought by menopause mixes up the hormonal cocktail in new and different proportions. As the levels of the primary female hormone, estrogen, continually decline, the chaser of male hormone, testosterone, increases in ratio. Before menopause, the average woman's level of testosterone is roughly 300 picograms. After a woman goes through the Change, if her ovaries are still intact, her testosterone level falls from 300 to about 215-220—or one-third. (If her ovaries are removed, the drop is to about 100, or a two-thirds fall.) At the same time, her estrogen level falls twelve-fold, a far greater decrease than that in the male hormone. And after the Change, her estrogen level remains fairly constant.

Therefore, the balance between female and male hormones is dramatically altered by menopause. "In a *pre*menopausal woman the ratio of testosterone to estrogen is roughly two to one, whereas in a *post*menopausal woman the ratio is roughly twenty to one," concludes Dr. Howard Judd, professor of Obstetrics and Gynecology at the University of California, Los Angeles (UCLA), whose scientific studies established these norms.

This provides a biological basis that would explain, at least in part, the widespread phenomenon of postmenopausal zest and the greater assertiveness recorded, cross-culturally, among postmenopausal women. Aggressiveness is rooted in the male hormone testosterone and found in elevated levels in men and male baboons of high rank.

Hence, in many societies, middle-aged women—freed from the role of breeder and fired up with relatively higher levels of testosterone—rise in rank and power, in political, religious, economic, and community life. Margaret Mead, a mentor of mine, summed it up in one sentence: "There is no greater power in the world than the zest of a postmenopausal woman."

Indeed, the most powerful woman in the world throughout the decade of the Eighties was a menopausal woman. Margaret Thatcher was just about fifty when she broke the glass ceiling in British politics and became leader of the Conservative Party. She went through menopause while making the leap to world leader. Eleanor Roosevelt, Golda Meir, and Indira Gandhi all came into their own in their postmenopausal years.

Today, many more women are rising to high levels in public life in Europe and America, and without having to be honorary males. The American Secretary of State, Madeleine Albright, and Attorney General Janet Reno, the first woman to hold the post of top law enforcement officer in the U.S., are prime examples of strong-minded women with plenty of postmenopausal zest. Among the women in the European Parliament are some very glamorous women. Twenty-nine of the fifty-four political women who were elected to the U.S. Congress in 1992 were in their fifties or over. Across Europe and North America there seems to be a new recognition: You don't have to be old and gray and male to be knowledgeable. You can be fifty and female and fearless.

It would be remiss of me to represent all contemporary women in their middle years as similarly enlightened. Indeed, some of those with readiest access to the facts of life about the postmenopausal years are the most confused by the politicized debate over HRT.

Any honest examination of the hormonal differences between women and men—or between women and other women, for that matter—is dismissed by writers like Barbara Ehrenreich as a surrender to the old biology-as-destiny credo. The cessation of menses, she wants us to believe, is "an obvious nonevent." (Like puberty?) Menopause isn't an event at all, but a *process* that takes place over five to seven years and has as many profound metaphysical, social, and sexual layers of meaning as the passage of menarche, which ushers in a woman's fertility.

These polemicists seriously misrepresent the movement to bring menopause out of the closet. Beware of this logic when you encounter it. The proponents are often women frozen in an outdated era of feminism. Ignoring a host of new data that demonstrate some clear gender differences stemming, at least in part, from variations in male/female biology, they represent their views as a higher good than the truth. It can make them more dangerous than the wrong drug.

Menopause
in the
Workplace

❦

$\mathcal{T}$he boardrooms of America are lighting up with hot flashes. So many of the "point women" among baby boomers—those now in their mid-forties to fifties who are the first among their generation to approach the passage into menopause—are already operating at 110 percent. They may be in command positions in their professional lives, poised to crash through the glass ceiling. Or they may be completing a suspended college education, starting over to get a graduate degree, or launching a new business. Those who have remained childless may now be eager to adopt or to turn their care-giving instincts into a renewed form of social obligation. The married women have a new chance for romance with a neglected husband, if the nest is now empty. Those divorced or widowed may choose to savor their independence or delight in a new love, or a new sexual orientation. The openings are numerous for women today as they enter their Flaming Fifties.

But at the same time, many are likely to be sand-wiched between an abruptly dependent parent or in-law who is entering the twilight of ill health and the continued dependence of children who are still likely to be living at home today, and who, well into their twenties, consider it their prerogative to move back in! This is no time suddenly to find that one can't sleep, can't shake the blues, or can't call up facts memorized the day before.

Sylvia Chase, a correspondent for ABC's *Prime Time Live* and a pioneer since 1971 in network TV, remembers all too vividly trying to deal with meno-pause in the workplace. "I had a hysterectomy, and about a year later menopause hit me. There was some perception around the network that I was in 'poor health.' After consulting many colleagues, I took my superior, a male executive, to lunch. I explained that I had juvenile diabetes, so the hysterectomy had been a difficult operation. I went on and on with a very patient explanation. Finally, I said, 'Are there any more questions, because I'd like to get this all out in the open so my health isn't an issue.' He was a very mature, very smart man, but he was probably so embarrassed that he changed the subject to something classically sexist.

" 'So, are you and so-and-so still an item?' " he asked.

Chase thought to herself, *God, did I make any progress here?*

Progress has been slow, but as menopause is more and more candidly discussed in medical, social, and political environments, it is also beginning to be addressed in the workplace. As a result of the wom-en's movement, midlife women are firmly ensconced in all levels of the work force. Many college-educated women now in their fifties took jobs after being left economically strapped by divorce or by a husband who was downsized, underemployed, or who retired early. Once they felt the stimulation and boost in self-esteem so often provided by working for one's own paycheck, many saw their horizons expand. They may plan to continue working for many years.

About 80 percent of the nearly three million American woman aged 50 to 60 who graduated from college are in the work force today.

Employment among all women in their fifties, educated or not, has also risen steeply in the last decade to 8.1 million, or 65 percent of this age group (up from 54 percent in 1984), according to new data collected by the Labor Department. And here is the grand sweep: When the millenium turns, about nineteen million women will be in the prime menopause age span of forty-five to fifty-four, according to projections by *American Demographics*. And by that time women will make up fully half the labor force.

These striking statistics are the result of the last thirty years of struggle by women to secure their place in every form of employment—whether in blue-collar jobs or in corporate boardrooms. It seems a cruel irony that some who now enjoy their positions may lose their confidence because of the temporary or untreated disruptions of menopause, which can interrupt a woman's job performance without warning, depending on the severity of her symptoms. For some it can even put their livelihood at risk.

Constanza is a case in point. A fixture at the

cashier's stool in a busy hospital cafeteria, Constanza had received consistently positive reviews for many years in the same job. Suddenly, tearfully, at fifty-two, she announced she was leaving. Due to downsizing and consolidation, her position had become more multi-tasked. Not only did she have to work the register, she also had to make sandwiches at the sandwich bar. It was too much, she couldn't cope. When she quit, her boss said, "You're a good employee, let's try again." But she was so frustrated and upset with herself that she walked out. On her exit interview, she admitted that she was crying a lot after work. "I'm just having an awful time with menopause," she said.

For women in high-level executive positions who are dealing with menopause, there can be special challenges. "Many symptoms are simply nuisances, but for women in power, symptoms such as great variations in energy can be very disturbing, as can forgetfulness or lack of focus," says Dr. Patricia Allen.

"It's difficult for anyone to try to function after a string of sleepless nights," concurs Dr. Lila Nachtigall, director of the Women's Wellness Division at New York University Medical School. "It's a hundred times worse if you have fifty people reporting to you, four deadlines and a plane to catch in an hour."

Sharon, the head of her own diversified company, is a woman of forty-nine who travels the globe scouting new business. She has always depended on her instant recall of telephone numbers and memos dictated on the run. Seemingly overnight, as her cycles became erratic, so did her concentration and short-term memory. "I began to be terrified that I would be holding a meeting and simply wouldn't be able to think fast on my feet," she confided to me when we shared a plane ride. Her doctor had no answers. She had begun to consider seriously whether or not to sell her business before she failed it.

Shortly thereafter, at my suggestion, she attended a women's health symposium and realized she was in the stormy portion of an otherwise temporary passage. That calmed her down and she began shepherding her energies more intelligently. Other executives were trained to take on some of the traveling. Sharon became fiercely disciplined about getting a decent night's sleep, counteracting jet lag with naps, and giving herself time off for yoga and therapeutic massages. Soon, she was back on her game.

Two points are imperative to keep in mind:

First, the vast majority of women do not have all the symptoms described herein. Some have almost no symptoms. And most have a modest, relatively manageable experience of menopausal phenomena.

Secondly, most symptoms diminish in a matter of months, or maybe a year or so, and over time disappear altogether, or disappear immediately with hormone replacement therapy. This process can be accelerated by making lifestyle changes, such as regular exercising and the diet and herbal remedies (see p. 88).

Human Resource Professionals on the Front Lines

✑

*N*ot surprisingly, many women professionals are cautious about bringing menopause "out of the closet" at the workplace, for fear of opening a Pandora's box that could create a political backlash. June Fisher, manager of employee relations at Mary Hitchcock Memorial Hospital in Lebanon, New Hampshire, has heard this fear expressed by more than a few of the eight hundred women between the ages of forty and fifty-five who work at the hospital. "One female employee was very concerned about anything that might suggest that we're different or unable to compete with men," she said. "Another woman warned, 'This could be a double-edged sword. Be careful with it. We've worked so hard, we don't want to give the impression that menopausal women can't keep it together."

Educating management—and women themselves—about menopause will be key to working through the barriers. The model is already in place. It wasn't so long ago that pregnancy held back women in being hired or advanced, until legal protections were put in place and the consciousness of employers and employees alike was raised. Today, visibly pregnant women continue in their roles as TV anchors, bus drivers, political candidates. There are signs that small inroads are being made to introduce the subject of menopause through employee seminars and workshops, but major obstacles still exist.

"The experience of menopause is not really a workplace obstacle for a career woman; it's *other people's* response to it," says Susan Sangillo Bellifemine, senior vice president and senior counsel for Prudential Securities. "If we remove the veil of secrecy around the issue, people may be comfortable talking about it in the workplace. An atmosphere of secrecy can increase anxiety. An open discussion may result in more tolerance. And not only by men, but by those non-menopausal women who refuse to accept the inevitability of the Change."

The denial of menopause by unsympathetic female coworkers creates a particularly painful challenge for women who are struggling with a severe degree of symptoms. A woman I'll call "Marcia," a forty-eight-year-old studio technician at a TV station in San Francisco, placed her trust in a female colleague about ten years younger, thinking it safe to share with a younger girlfriend her ongoing struggle with menopause and hormone replacement therapy.

"[Later at work] I reacted to something in a more assertive way than I normally would—some little screwup," recalls Marcia. "A male cameraman just laughed and said, 'Oh, shut up and take your hormones!' Since I had recently mentioned hormones to my female colleague, I immediately felt, 'Oh no, she spilled the beans.' I was just mortified. I didn't know how to respond."

June Fisher has seen repeated instances of this sort of sniping among women at her hospital. "There's an attitude that the woman has some control over the process [of menopause]—that she can take a pill so that she doesn't show her symptoms. Unfortunately, it's women—especially women of the same age who did *not* experience a difficult menopause—who feel this way."

In the spring of 1997, a symposium chaired by Dr. Patricia Allen and myself entitled "Menopause in the Workplace," was held under the auspices of The New York Menopause Research Foundation and the Cornell Lecture Series. One hundred human resource administrators attended the conference. Although many of these front-line professionals were cautious about opening up the subject of menopause at their own places of business, most thought it was inevitable and important.

"Not enough women have an understanding of how menopause is affecting both their work and private lives. Lots of women are also uneducated about the very prolonged perimenopausal phase and its effects," said one respondent.

The one hundred professionals answered a survey on "Managing Menopause in the Workplace." Only 9 percent said their companies offered any programs to educate staff or management about male or female menopause, or how to cope with any life-stage changes. Yet, 80 percent believed their companies or organizations would benefit from enhanced productivity by valued employees if they took a proactive approach to educating management and employees about menopause.

But even the benefits of education come with a cautionary note. "Heightening awareness of this issue in the workplace must be done with great care lest 'What if she's menopausal?' replaces 'What if she gets pregnant?'" warned another participant.

"Any human resource officer at this point in time has to be aware that in the workplace, we are going to have a huge number of women experiencing menopause, and they need to know all they can about it," warns June Fisher of Mary Hitchcock Memorial Hospital. "If they don't, they're going to have employee relations situations that they're not going to recognize, like not seeing a train coming down the track."

Menopausal health problems do not yet entitle an employee to any legal protections. In order to qualify for protection under the Family Medical Leave Act (FMLA), one must exhibit a very high level of disability, as well as certification from a physician. To date, the FMLA has *not* been invoked in connection with menopause-related symptoms. FMLA experts, however, do *not* rule it out as a possibility in the future.

Menopausal women are learning what they can do for themselves when it comes to handling hot flashes or intense perspiring while at a meeting, interacting with customers, or delivering a speech from a lectern. When the subject is discussed openly among women, they have an opportunity to share some of their own solutions, such as bringing a change of clothes to work in case of an uncontrollable drenching or a hair dryer to repair dripping wet hair.

It is important to emphasize the added value that a postmenopausal woman brings to the workplace. She is no longer haunted by child care problems that can drive her crazy at work. "I'd much prefer hiring a postmenopausal woman than one who is in the throes of dating or one who is distracted by understandable concerns and chaos of childrearing," was the candid admission of a top human resources director who attended our conference. Postmenopausal women show up on time, and their professionalism and sophistication allows them to become team leaders and to serve as mentors to younger employees. They know how the world works and are usually no longer fazed by petty office politics. In most cases, the postmenopausal woman is a dream employee.

While passing through menopause might bring doubt and difficulties, it is a bridge to the second half of life—a potential Second Adulthood often ushered in by a flourish of new vitality. Many women report feeling more confident, empowered, involved, and energized than in their earlier years.

This is not news to some ancient cultures. It is the women in their 50s, 60s, 70s and beyond who are among the most industrious members of a northern Tanzanian tribe studied by Dr. Kristen Hawkes of the University of Utah. She found that these women, of the Hadza tribe, unburdened by the duties of childrearing, are out in the woods seven or eight hours a day gathering food for their community. Older women also play the role of the doting grandmother, helping to raise the tribe's children while the younger women are busy nursing and cannot fend for their families. These hard-working grandmothers are, in fact, central to the survival of the tribe.

"The Grandmother Hypothesis gives us a whole new way of understanding why modern humans suddenly were able to go everywhere and do everything," says Dr. Hawkes. "It may explain why we took over the planet."

Dr. Hawkes and her colleagues suggest that the extension of life past menopause was a watershed event in human prehistory, eventually affecting the labor force. With elder females available for tending the children, adults were then free to colonize new territories inaccessible to those primates that could not leave their young and forage new areas. In today's world, for those older women who find themselves in the work force, creative solutions must be sought to make their menopausal and postmenopausal years just as productive as primitive tribeswomen's.

The
Perimenopause
Panic

✣

$\mathcal{W}$e can now break down the menopausal transition into several distinctly different phases. The first phase—*perimenopause*—is the least understood and potentially most confusing and symptomatic. Perimenopause is the months or years of transition from the childbearing years to the complete cessation of menstrual cycles that is menopause. Women enter this transition some time between forty and fifty. Yet the vast majority of women have no idea they are in something called "perimenopause." It is the most confusing phase, when hormonal fluctuations are the most volatile and when women experience the greatest number of symptoms compared with any other stage.

The spectrum of signs and symptoms in perimenopause is bafflingly broad. One woman will brush it off—"I feel hot for a few seconds a couple of times a day, but not enough to bother me"—while another is terrified that she will flare purple and start leaking drops of perspiration during another business conference or forget phone numbers she just looked up. A third woman, who complains of waking up four or five times a night, swamped in sweat, changing nightgowns, having Thermostat Wars with her husband, is mistakenly diagnosed as being in clinical depression. In truth, she is suffering from the effects of serious sleep deprivation.

It hardly seems possible that these people are all talking about the same organic process.

So far, there has not been much research on perimenopause, and only recently have physicians begun to recognize perimenopause as a distinct stage before actual menopause. A woman's attitude and awareness going into this first phase of the silent passage have a profound impact on how it is experienced.

Entering perimenopause is very much like entering puberty. It is reminiscent of the first time one got one's period—the I-could-die feeling when a girlfriend whispered, "You have a spot on the back of your skirt," and you had to back out of the glee club rehearsal so no one would see. And now, at the dignified apex of one's adulthood, to have to worry about being hit with surprise periods or hot flashes, night sweats and insomnia, sudden bouts of waistline bloat, possibly heart palpitations, crying for no reason or temper outbursts, maybe migraines, incontinence, itchy, crawly skin, memory lapses—my God, what's going on?

In fact, menopause is much like puberty in that it does not happen in a "single moment." The sexual attraction associated with puberty, for instance, may first manifest itself as early as age nine or ten. The hormone charged with stirring things up so early is

DHEA, a powerful sex and growth hormone responsible for surges of development at birth and age six, reaching adult levels around eighteen.

When does perimenopause begin? For former First Lady Barbara Bush's generation of mostly nonworking wives, it was around age fifty. Contemporary women should expect the first signs much earlier. The latest surveys reveal a surprising number of women in their *early forties* are perimenopausal. Researchers admit they have underestimated the number of younger women who experience all the symptoms of menopause even though they still have periods.

There is a difference between perimenopause and premature ovarian failure. The average age of menopause is fifty, plus or minus seven years, and it is clinically defined as not having a menstrual period for a whole year. Premature ovarian failure can be genetic, or surgical (from a hysterectomy where ovaries are also removed), or chemical—that is from chemotherapy. "Premature menopause isn't any more common today than it ever has been," says Dr. Howard Zacur of Johns Hopkins Hospital. "But so many women in their late thirties and early forties are suffering from perimenopausal symptoms," they may think they are in premature menopause.

Some researchers contend that perimenopause starts around age thirty-seven or thirty-eight, when the ovaries begin to lose egg-producing follicles at an accelerating rate. Others suggest that it comes later, when the spacing between periods starts to deviate from one's normal pattern.

Early Signs

❦

It is during perimenopause—in their forties—that women feel most estranged from their bodies. Half of all women who have hot flashes will begin feeling them while they are still menstruating normally, starting as early as age forty. Studies show that most women have hot flashes for two years. One quarter of women have them for five years. And 10 percent have them for the rest of their lives.

The first sign of perimenopause is very often *not* hot flashes but gushing: a sudden heavy flow of blood that may be dark or clotted and that may seep through the normal protection. Your cycle will get longer or shorter, lighter or heavier, closer together or farther apart. This is all normal. Almost everybody bleeds erratically during perimenopause. It happens when we stop ovulating every month. The months when ovulation doesn't occur, we produce no progesterone—the hormone ordinarily responsible for flushing the lining of the uterus. The endometrial lining becomes thicker and may not be entirely discarded until the next cycle, when the body rids itself of the previous buildup.

One month a woman may have a heavy period, another month nothing; all of a sudden she may develop cysts in her breast, or functional ovarian cysts, and two months or a year later she may be back to normal. The reason for all the volatility is that hormone levels are surging and falling in frantic response to desperate signals from the brain to the pituitary. Her menstrual cycle not only becomes erratic but is uncoupled from her temperature and sleep cycles, and these disruptions of basic body functions affect her appetite, sexual interest, and overall sense of well-being. The body's whole balance is thrown off.

Ellen McGrath, who was named 1997 psychologist of the year by the American Psychological Association, says, "I'm seeing younger women whose doctors deny that they are having menopausal kinds of experiences or hormonal fluctuations. You have this huge population of women in their early forties who are having these experiences, and a huge medical establishment denying it is anything other than 'psychological' because it doesn't fit the classic definition of menopause."

Phyllis Mansfield, an academic researcher at Pennsylvania State University who studies female cycles, registered the first signs of the Change in herself in her early forties. Having always had a normal and very predictable cycle, she was unnerved when her periods became heavier and more frequent. "I would have to schedule family camping trips and conferences around my cycle." Although she studied and went for checkups, still, in the back of her mind, was a common fear: *Are my organs deteriorating?*

"I'd have a really long period of magnificent energy and acute mental functioning, even brilliance, when I'm never tired, always very up, producing like crazy. At first I thought, *Oh! So this is going to be part of my new personality.* Then just as suddenly I fell into a period of intense anxiety—and that lasted for a month. I thought, *So, is this it?* But once I got my period, the despondency just lifted and dissipated in one day. So then you think, *What happens when there are no more cycles? Is there one mood that persists? Is it permanent mellowing? Permanent anything?"*

While this can be very unsettling, the important thing to know is this:

Perimenopause is a temporary phenomenon.

Best Defenses

❧

It is a time to plan to reduce stressful pressures wherever possible and to pamper yourself a little bit. But there is no reason to panic or drive yourself into a frenzy looking for the perfect "cure." Resistance to accepting that one has entered the long passage leading out of youth and fertility and into unfamiliar territory is perfectly understandable. But remaining resistant to that reality blocks a woman from entering her Second Adulthood.

As a practitioner in New York City, Dr. Patricia Allen has observed over the past several years that the former silence about menopause has turned into an obsession. "Baby boom women come into my office now in an information-feeding frenzy," she says. "They want the perfect treatment without consequences." She tells women, "It is important that you make informed choices. But you also have to recognize that everything we do, or don't do, has some price."

Women who don't want to rush to take hormones, or who can't for health reasons, have many milder ways to counteract the symptoms of perimenopause. For example, a feisty British-American woman who works out regularly at my health club and looks about sixteen was shocked when she began waking up several times a night all hot and sweaty. Being British, she leaned toward homeopathic remedies. "So I just doubled up on my Vitamin E (from 400 to 800 I.U.) and my evening primrose oil and my Royal Jelly. My gynecologist said it can't hurt me, and I'm sleeping again."

Restoring restful sleep is probably the number one priority for most women in a symptomatic perimenopause. This is the ideal time to practice meditation, to learn the relaxation response that counteracts anxiety, or to take up yoga and learn how to breathe from the diaphragm.

Other natural remedies for perimenopausal symptoms are becoming more well-known. Dong quai, the Chinese herb, contains plant sterols that have estrogenlike effects. Plant estrogens are estimated to be one four-hundredth as strong as the estrogen from pregnant mare's urine found in Premarin. Dong quai is available in health food stores in capsules, liquid, black beans, or tea form. Black cohosh is the other most effective supplement. Vitamin E and licorice are old faithfuls. Siberian ginseng is possibly helpful in opposing fatigue and depressive symptoms. It, too, is available in health food stores, or easily taken as ginseng tea. (See chapter "Partnering Yourself Through a Natural Menopause.") Adding frequent helpings of tofu or soy milk, both of which contain a high degree of plant estrogens, is a mild and safe way to rebalance your body at this stage.

But what about the long-term changes that might not be announced by any symptoms until it is too late?

Silent Changes

$\mathcal{T}$he acceleration of bone loss also begins during the perimenopausal phase, as do other changes in the long-term health status of the older woman. "The problem is, nobody *feels* the bone they're losing until it's too late," says Dr. Robert Lindsay. "That is, osteoporosis is without symptoms until it becomes disease."

We build all the bone we are going to make by the time we're thirty-five. "Women really start to lose bone mass at forty," says Richard Bockman, head of the endocrine department and codirector of the Osteoporosis Center at the Hospital for Special Surgery in Manhattan. "Bone loss occurs rapidly even before the menopause, then accelerates during the menopause as hormones fall off, and eventually tapers off to a slower rate of loss about ten years after the onset of menopause." Generally, this timetable of bone loss occurs in all white women, according to the National

Osteoporosis Foundation in Washington, D.C., though not necessarily for women of color.

Similarly, silent changes in the blood vessels that nourish the heart begin taking place during perimenopause. Estrogen makes a woman's blood vessels more elastic. Nature provides this relaxing hormone in abundance during the reproductive years because whenever a woman is pregnant, her blood volume expands. If her blood vessels were as rigid as a man's, the increase in blood pressure would kill both mother and fetus in about the fifth month, according to Dr. Estelle Ramey, professor emeritus and physiologist at Georgetown University.

"So all during your young years, whether you get pregnant or not, you walk around with more elastic blood vessels—until menopause," says Dr. Ramey. When a woman stops producing estrogen, her good cholesterol (HDL) level falls. Bad (LDL) cholesterol levels start increasing during the transition *into* menopause, as confirmed by the National Institutes of Health. Thus begins for women the narrowing of arteries that will gradually expose them to the cardiovascular disease from which estrogen protected them during their fertile years.

In addition to noticing a lessening of lubrication in the vagina, many women notice bladder problems or suffer the embarrassment of feeling a sudden urge to urinate before they can make it to the bathroom. This "urge incontinence" is common, though little discussed, and may be associated with lack of estrogen. Also, the uterus changes shape as women get older and may come to press on the organs of the urinary tract. Male urologists usually shun female patients with such chronic complaints. There may be no more than fifty female urologists in the United States. One of them, Dr. Suzanne Frye in Manhattan, says the problem is easily correctable in most cases. A drug called Ditropan can reverse this bladder instability and change a menopausal woman's life.

"But I have cystic breasts, so I can't take hormones, right?" women would often ask in the group interviews. Cystic breasts are not uncommon at this stage. Dr. Hiram Cody, one of the top breast surgeons at New York Hospital, explains, "During the perimenopausal period breasts can become lumpier and more tender than before, due to surges of excess estrogen. It subsides within a year after periods stop."

Should women who are suffering the worst symptoms of menopause and accelerated health deficits be able to start hormone replacement therapy during perimenopause? The old dogma said no. Dr. Allen summarizes current practice.

"We know now that there are good medical reasons for some women to begin hormone replacement therapy during the perimenopause years. Acceleration of bone loss begins, risks for coronary artery disease start to increase, atrophy of breast and genital tissue starts. And so, most doctors now believe that a woman who is bothered by menopausal symptoms, if she chooses HRT, should be treated before the cessation of her periods."

According to Howard Zacur, M.D., Ph.D., director of the Johns Hopkins Estrogen Consultation Service, recognizing perimenopause as a distinct stage before actual menopause is essential in order to provide the correct medical treatment. The type of hormone replacement therapy given to women in true menopause is not sufficient to halt perimenopausal symptoms, he says. During perimenopause the body still manufactures its own estrogen, erratically, now and then causing an excess of the hormone. "The way around it is to give a dose of estrogen high enough to suppress the body from making its own, such as that contained in oral contraceptive pills."

Low-dose oral contraceptives deal with the continuing risk of pregnancy even as they alleviate hot flashes and irregular or heavy bleeding.

Dancing Around
Depression

❧

"*I* think I'm going crazy" was a frightened admission Dr. Morris Notelovitz frequently heard at the Women's Health Center in Gainesville, Florida, where he saw extreme cases. "Many women feel it's very difficult to concentrate. They can hear what's going on, they know they're there, but it's as though their body is just witnessing." These are women whose hormones are falling and spiking and falling again, six times a day or even a half dozen times within an hour. They feel—and, in fact, they are— out of control of their bodies. They may also feel at the mercy of erratic moods. Is it all in their minds?

Whether or not depression is associated with menopause has been a subject of intense debate, mostly because of a looseness of terminology and the Freudian hangover. Freud related the loss of reproductive potential with mourning and involutional melancholia. Indeed, it was common in our mothers' day for women in the Change to be institutionalized. "Ner-

vous breakdown" it was called, because nobody associated their intense if temporary depression with the
temporary breakdown of hormonal balance.

The mood swings so characteristic of perimenopause may bring on sadness, malaise, mild depression, irritability, poor concentration—in general, the
feeling of being on a roller coaster. Western medicine
still fosters the erroneous assumption that these *temporary* mental symptoms herald a marked deterioration in the mental health of postmenopausal women.
Exactly the opposite is true. It is women in their mid-
to-late forties who manifest a peak in minor mental
symptoms in the five years *immediately prior* to the
end of their cycles. Something changes profoundly
between the years of entry to this passage and the
completion of it, when the hallmark is a euphoric
burst of new energy. Studies now confirm that women
in the *post*-menopausal years show *less* evidence of
any psychological problems than younger women.

Yet outmoded cultural attitudes swing tremendous
weight in influencing how a woman copes at this time
of life. Seeking to correct this oversight, Dr. C.B.
Ballinger, an eminent Scottish psychiatrist, academic
researcher, and consultant at Royal Dundee Liff Hospital, found in a review of recent British and Dutch
population surveys that "complaints of 'mental imbalance,' fatigue, depression, and irritability were
most common in women who were still menstruating
and reached a peak . . . in women reporting irregular
menstrual periods who could be considered immediately premenopausal." Ballinger's own study confirmed that it was the women aged forty-five to
forty-nine years *and still menstruating* who had the
highest levels of negative mental effects. But she then

followed up and found from population surveys that "women in the postmenopausal years show less evidence of psychiatric disturbance than younger women." Her conclusions are consistent with those reached by several other researchers using very different survey techniques.

The much-publicized Massachusetts Women's Health Study reported in a 1986 Harvard Medical School publication that "depression in middle-aged women is associated mainly with events and circumstances unrelated to the hormonal changes that occur at menopause." Epidemiologist Sonja McKinlay, co-author of the study with her husband, John, insisted, "Most women just go straight through menopause, no problem. None, nor with irritability."

Try out that line on a room full of menopausal-aged women and one is guaranteed a laugh. The McKinlays' conclusion—that depression at this stage is associated *only* with external "social circumstances"—was suspect since it was a paper-and-pencil questionnaire and no measurements had been taken of the actual hormone levels in peri- and postmenopausal women.

Alice Lawrence, forty-five, a nurse from Carolina Beach, North Carolina, saw the first signs of menopause at age thirty-five. "I attributed my mood changes to stress—my mother was ill and I was going back to school for my RN—but I was still in denial. I had what I call my 'Meno Rages.' I would get so pissed off that I wanted to hear bones break and glass shatter. It was like a temper tantrum but I would always cry after the raging part was over. I would sometimes even get on the floor and curl up and cry. I felt so horrible, so ugly, so dastardly inside." Her malaise, although frightening at the time, lifted within several months.

It is true that *clinical* depression subsides in women over fifty. And irritability and depression in middle-aged women do have many other sources. But mood changes are so commonly mentioned by women in the perimenopause phase, why should women be told there is no hormonal basis for feeling depressed?

Dr. Howard Fillit, a gerontologist at Mount Sinai Hospital in New York City, describes a common misconception: "A woman comes into a doctor's office at age fifty-one with the menopause and says, 'Doctor, I can't function very well in the office. I think I have memory loss, I can't pay attention to my work, and I feel really depressed.' The doctor looks at major depression as a disease. The literature tells him there's no major association of depression with the menopause, so he says, 'C'mon, you're crazy.' If the doctor was aware that these complaints and symptoms are real, although they may not qualify as a disease, this problem could be dealt with in a constructive manner."

In fact, estrogen does improve mood and the sense of psychological well-being even in well-adjusted women who have no distressing menopausal symptoms, according to a study done by Dr. Edward Ditkoff at the University of Southern California School of Medicine. Women in the random study who were given the standard dose of 0.625 mg of estrogen a day showed a decided improvement in depression scores and were more optimistic and confident than those given placebos. Neurobiologically estrogen has chemical effects on the brain that are similar to antidepressants. The most experienced researchers say that when estrogen levels in the blood are very low, a woman might start to feel a bit sad or blue or notice irritability or mood swings, but not of a clinical magnitude.

That is the key distinction: Women low in estrogen often have feelings of malaise, as opposed to suffering from the textbook definition of depression as disease (the criteria used in the McKinlays' Massachusetts study). Unless there are also underlying causes, the blues that may color the years leading up to menopause are a temporary phenomenon.

Two areas of behavior have been found by Dr. Ballinger to be very widely influenced by menopause: Sleep and sexual response. Indeed, one of the most common sources of mood changes at this stage of life is broken sleep. Night sweats that awaken a woman several times, interrupting REM sleep night after night, can easily produce all the consequences of sleep deprivation. A major function of REM sleep is to allow important brain cells to rest and replenish their chemical stores, according to the latest dream research at Harvard Medical School. It also releases sleep-promoting transmitters and is crucial in regulating body temperature. So it should come as no surprise that a person awakened by temperature aberrations, and deprived of the REM sleep needed to reset the body's thermostat, is stuck in a vicious circle.

"These are real symptoms. Don't think you're crazy," Dr. Robert Lindsay tells his patients. A good-humored Scottish-born endocrinologist, Lindsay was asked by New York State to set up a bone center in conjunction with Columbia University. His clinic at the Helen Hayes Bone Center is now booked almost a year in advance because, he says, women are not getting reasonable answers to their questions about menopause elsewhere. "The reason estrogen works so well in curing menopausal depression is that it restores REM sleep," he says. "Once women can sleep better, they're fine. They don't need a psychiatrist or a divorce."

Indeed, the best place for a woman to get help on mood and stage-of-life questions during this transition—provided she has no history of depression, alcohol or drug dependency, and isn't suffering from horrific hot flashes—is not to medicalize her menopause, but to get into a support group and learn from other women.

From the Pits
to the Peak

Women I have interviewed often describe a "pit" or "low" during their mid-to-late forties, complicated in many cases by the confusing symptoms of perimenopause. In the course of research for my recent book, *New Passages: Mapping Your Life Across Time,* I did national surveys of over seven thousand women. Those with the poorest sense of well-being were, on average, forty-seven years old—the pits. But it comes back strong in the early fifties. Those enjoying the highest sense of well-being *compared to any other stage of their lives* were fifty-three—the peak.

Facing the entryway of any new major passage in the life cycle is always far more daunting than actually moving through the transition. So many women in *post*menopause have described to me, sometimes with bemused amazement, how vital and energetic and *focused* they feel. I was amused myself when I had a late lunch recently with a male friend in his mid-fifties. After walking thirty city blocks to the restaurant, I found my companion already halfway through his soup. "I just couldn't wait," he said. "You're still going strong and you probably got up at six o'clock this morning."

I was taken aback. "How did you know?"

"Because women your age always seem to get up at six in the morning. You're more energetic than ever— just at the time we men are starting to wind down." He was right about that switch, generally speaking, but such a comforting perspective is not real or believable for women until they themselves have actually come through the Change.

The passage of menopause is inextricably bound up with other common life events and cultural determinants. Harsh losses such as a parent's life-threatening illness or death are new and real around this time. The inescapable evidence of physical aging and the cruel penalties of ageism also register. Women are brutally premature in disqualifying *themselves* as no longer attractive to men, simply because they are no longer young. And there is the artifact of generation. Many pre-Boomer women were not prepared, professionally or emotionally, for the reality that being an earner becomes central to the self-esteem—and often the survival—of women in the middle years. The shift in body chemistry may be a casual matter compared with the faltering of one's former identity as the role of mother becomes distant and custodial, if not outright rejected. The menopausal identity crisis is exaggerated if one begins at the same time to lose social contact through divorce, retirement, or widowhood.

Disengagement from the mothering role along with the end of fertility, however, turn out to be precursors to the beneficent change in body chemistry and mental outlook summed up in the term "postmenopausal zest."

So, despite the danger zone through which most women will pass in their late forties, a mobilization usually begins shortly after menopause, and a profound change in self-concept begins to register with rising exhilaration for many women as they move into their fifties. They often break the seal on repressed angers. They overcome the habits of trying to be perfect and of needing to make everyone love them. They may shed the terror of living without a man that trapped them in a dead or destructive marriage. Many women, during the decade of the mid-forties to the mid-fifties, find the sustained courage to extricate themselves from lives of desperate repetition.

The sense of well-being is more than happiness, the latter generally conveying relief from pent-up frustration or deprivation. Well-being registers deep in our unconscious, as a sustained background tone of equanimity—a calm, composed sense of all-rightness—that remains behind the more intense contrasts of daily events, including periods of unhappiness.

Several caveats must be added to these generalized statements on depression and menopause. Depression *is* correlated with surgical menopause. Most women feel relieved immediately after a hysterectomy. But a review of research by psychologist Ellen McGrath, editor of the American Psychological Association's 1990 task force report on *Women and Depression,* shows that women who have had hysterectomies are twice as likely to become depressed over time. The impact on sexual responsiveness and desire may be a major culprit. It is also likely that a woman who has suffered from phases of depression in the past will react in the same way during the transition of menopause.

The Massachusetts study confirms these observations. The two groups of women found most likely to become depressed are those who have experienced depression prior to menopause and women who have had hysterectomies. "Depression is associated with surgical menopause, but it may be the cause rather than the consequence of the surgery since the group of women who undergo hysterectomies is atypical," reports the study. Among those who were found on follow-up to have had the highest rates of depression, usually during perimenopause (apart from those with hysterectomies), were widowed, divorced, and separated women with less than twelve years of education. Never-married women showed the lowest rates of depression. Married women fell between the two extremes.

Women who are used to having mood swings with PMS appear to be very sensitive to hormonal fluctuation. "It has been observed that women who have had emotional problems during earlier times of hormonal change will probably have them again during menopause," says Dr. Jeanne L. Leventhal, clinical assistant professor of psychiatry at Stanford School of Medicine. Again there is good news: Such women experience great relief when they reach the *post*menopausal period. They are released from the treacherous mood baths of their reproductive years and feel a consistency of calmness at last.

"Stress Menopause"

❧

*I*t used to be that a reliable guide to when you might expect menopause is when your mother experienced it. But the mothers of today's groundbreaking women knew nothing like the level of workplace stress and environmental toxins we live with today. Acute or prolonged stress has been shown to increase the severity of symptoms in phase one of menopause and may even precipitate it prematurely. In fact, severe stress can reduce ovarian function and precipitate a temporary menopause at any time from the late thirties on. It may happen around the time of death of a close relative or other traumatic events. The phenomenon is similar to that experienced by a college student up against exams who misses a period.

An anesthesiologist who deals with life and death every day, running an intensive care unit in a midwestern hospital, had her own life turned upside down in her fortieth year.

"I had a fire in my home that was rather devastating," she recounts. Having outstripped her own ex-pectations, she was habituated to a high-performance life. "Of course, I said, oh, well, it was just a fire. I lived in a hotel for six months with two children to care for and continued working very hard—there was my team to run at the hospital—and I was deter-mined that the fire would not have any impact on my life. It was just 'pedal to the metal' and go right on."

Noticing she was a little frantic, the anesthesiologist began vigorously exercising an hour or two daily, in addition to her work and parenting responsibilities. She dropped down to a scrawny 105 pounds and couldn't sleep. "I was anxious and depressed, though I didn't acknowledge it. Suddenly my periods, which have never been that regular, weren't around at all. And when I did sleep, I was waking up five or six times a night and throwing the covers off." Her dentist husband said to her after a few weeks, "Well, honey, I think you're in menopause."

"What! I am only forty years old, of course I am not in menopause." But the very next day she did her blood test. "My FSH and LH were off the wall and my estrogen was very low," she was chagrined to discover. "It took me about five minutes to put an Estraderm patch on my behind [a means of delivering estrogen through the skin], and within three days I felt my old self again," continued the anesthesiologist. After a couple of months she stopped using the estrogen patch, and her hormone levels remained normal. "It seems I had a case of temporary menopause, due to much stress," the physician diagnosed herself after the fact. It might also have been precipitated by the extreme weight loss, as found in young marathon runners with no body fat. "In any case," she says, "I look upon that little visit of menopause as one of the greatest gifts that God has ever given me because it made me quite sympathetic to older women."

Everyone wants to be the person she was before. But your body is signaling that this is truly a Change of Life: You cannot put the same demands on it and expect it to be there for you whenever you have a period of high demand or unexpected stress. You cannot continue indefinitely being the same person as your younger self. To attempt it is the best way to precipitate depression.

Chemotherapy can also bring on a premature menopause. A head nurse at a major metropolitan hospital told me her personal story, which, sadly, is no longer unusual. "I was diagnosed with breast cancer when I was thirty-seven and I had a mastectomy and a year of chemotherapy. It was the chemotherapy—the drug Cytoxan—that caused ovarian failure."

The most unsettling aspect of this crisis period in the nurse's life was caused by her own—and her doctors'—ignorance about the impact of premature menopause. Known for her natural organizational skills and unflappable temperament, she had organized patient care in a high-demand environment for fifteen years. The untimely menopause caused her months of interrupted sleep and insomnia, along with mounting anxiety and feelings of depression.

"Suddenly, without any change of environment, my organization skills were compromised," noticed the nurse. "I was much slower. It was very troublesome." As soon as the reason became clear, medication corrected the problems. Some women are lucky, however. Once the chemotherapy is over they do resume cycling naturally. But not all doctors are aware of these complications.

Menopause Moms

❦

*W*omen having babies in their forties know they have departed from life cycle norms when they have to put on reading glasses to breast-feed.

As baby boomers have extended the time given to building their careers, the advent of motherhood has been pushed back. Perhaps their sense of eternal youth has contributed to the idea that they can wait until their late thirties or early forties to find themselves pregnant with their first child.

"I am the only self-avowed menopausal mother in my son's preschool," was the amusing confession of Marcia Wallace, an actress who has worked on *The Bob Newhart Show* and *The Simpsons*. Marcia has cultivated the zany image of her celebrity with a red corkscrew-curled mop and loud colors and chandelier-sized earrings. But what struck me were the consequences of reversed life stages that her story represents. A late bloomer, Marcia devoted her young years to pursuing her career and postponed the personal commitments usually made by a woman in her twenties until she reached her forties. She married for the first time at forty-three.

"I figured, by then, all I had left was one egg on a walker," Marcia quips. So she became an adoptive mother two years later. And a mere year after that— guess what? Marcia's new variant on women's life stages might be called The Compressed Life: marriage at forty-three, motherhood at forty-five, and menopause at forty-six.

A late *first* pregnancy can trigger an earlier menopause. A hotshot businesswoman who delivered her first child in her mid-forties found herself afterwards often drenched in sweat and gloomy. She told herself it must be postpartum depression (which is, indeed, rooted in the temporary depletion of estrogen following childbirth.) When the symptoms went on for two years, she began to wonder. But the last thing she would have done was to consult a doctor about menopause.

Her life became a maelstrom of role overload, marital strife, and eventually the failure of her own business and ensuing lawsuits. Always trying to do more, like so many women, she paid little attention to the needs of her body. When she began to have panic attacks and tearful outbursts over the least little setback, she sought out a Chinese medicine practitioner. The diagnosis: early menopause. She was stunned.

"I'm a young mother—how can you even think I'm an old lady in menopause!" she demanded.

The practitioner explained that the combined demands of a late pregnancy and stressful life events had taken a toll. Her metabolism had become very slow and her hormone level increasingly unbalanced. The depressed woman did not want to accept this reality. She insisted that her problems must be related to PMS, and that she'd always had them in milder form. She went on running on empty.

In contrast, there is a hardy breed of women who are able to postpone childbirth because of genetic good fortune. A recent study by Harvard researchers shows that women who give birth naturally to children in their forties live longer than those whose children are born before their fortieth birthday. The study, which examined women who lived to at least one hundred, concluded that women whose genes predispose them to a longer life also have a gene marker that predisposes them to be able to give birth later and postpone menopause.

"It really isn't the act of having a child but rather the ability to conceive and have a healthy pregnancy [after forty] that tends to be a marker for aging slowly. It's all inherited," said Ruth Fretts, an obstetrician and gynecologist at Harvard Medical School and one of the study's authors. "But having a child in your forties is relatively rare. Only three percent of all births take place in women who are forty years of age or older."

Delaying a first pregnancy can make some women feel as if they are racing against the menopause clock. If conception proves difficult, they might seek the assistance of an infertility specialist, which doesn't come cheap. Blood work, infertility drugs and office checkups can run hundreds, even thousands of dollars; in vitro insemination and medication can set back the hopeful mother-to-be more than *$12,000*.

But with advancing medical technology, a woman

needn't necessarily worry about even having a child *before* menopause. In 1997, a sixty-three-year-old California woman gave birth long after she had made the menopause passage by using a donor's egg. True, the woman had duped the fertility program, which had a cut-off age of fifty-five, but given the benefits of exercise and plastic surgery, it's getting harder and harder to tell a woman's age.

One of the latest scientific accomplishments occurred recently in Atlanta where human eggs were frozen, thawed, and fertilized, resulting in a successful twin pregnancy. Fertility clinics had long been able to freeze sperm and embryos, but they had been stymied by their inability to freeze eggs. The upshot of all this is that it could eventually make menopause as we know it obsolete. In effect, a woman could have her own babies at any age if she stores her eggs when she is young. It could also enable women who face chemotherapy, which can damage the ovaries, to save their eggs for later.

Sex and the Change-of-Life Lover

One subject women are least likely to bring up in connection with menopause is any change in sexual interest. The raging hormones of adolescence may suddenly become the *un*raging hormones of menopause. Or, it may go exactly the other way.

For example, a high-profile movie executive I know went through a major career move in her late forties, the sort of jump that inevitably kicks up gossip: *Was she fired?* One of her best friends warned her: "You know, this could be a very bad mark on your career because people will say, 'She's probably postmenopausal.' You lose your value."

"What are you saying!" The executive gasped in disbelief. "A dried-up, over-the-hill me? Do you really think that could be the perception out there?" From a distance, clad in a T-shirt, jeans, and Top-Siders, the slim blond woman could still be mistaken for fourteen.

"Well, you *are* getting older," warned the friend, probably projecting her own menopausal malaise.

"But what's amazing is that at age fifty I'm having the best sex I've ever had," the movie executive told me confidently. Following a recent divorce, "that part of me has suddenly come to life." What does this have to do with menopause? Everything. Here is a woman who associates sexual potency with power, just like the men who have been her mentors and models at the top of corporate life.

"I made up my mind I'm not going to lose this part," she said fervently. And within the next two years she came through menopause with the support of a sexy and sensitive male companion. The two found a mature level of relationship and went on to commit to sharing their lives.

In general, it can be said that women who enjoyed a lively sex life when they were younger are likely to go on enjoying—or missing—sex after menopause. Some psychoanalysts like Graciella Abelin-Sas, a member of the New York Psychoanalytic Institute, hear a common confession from their female patients over fifty: "I've never been as aware of my sexual urges in my whole life." Dr. Abelin says, "Women are ashamed of this. The myth of aging has conditioned them to believe that their sexuality should be going down the drain. They often feel that they are the exception, and they are embarrassed about being so sexual." As their mates' potency declines, or they become widowed or divorced, some women over fifty seen by psychiatrists are turning to homosexual relationships with other women, which they had never considered before. "The female mates are more loving, and more accepting of the physical changes," says Dr. Abelin.

"Most women after the menopause, if they're reasonably healthy and happy, do not experience a diminution in sex drive," says Dr. Ramey, the senior physiologist at Georgetown University. "But a very large number do—maybe 30 percent," she estimates, adding that the figures are unreliable because doctors don't ask women about their sex drive. "Since we're all living longer, this large number of women who face a diminished sex drive can be a very serious matter."

It is particularly startling for women who have always been sensual to find even slight changes in intimate pleasures they have taken for granted. Gayle Sand is a case in point. A slinky, sexy-looking California woman with great black Diana Ross hair, she flew all the way to Manhattan to have her bone density measured at the Osteoporosis Center at the Hospital for Special Surgery—that's how jittery she was about this thing called menopause.

"I've always been a person that's looked much younger than I actually was. Even now I don't think I look forty-nine years old, do I?" She leaned back in the mean metal institutional chair, attempting a seductive nonchalance, and let the strap of her laminated white tank top drop off one deeply tanned shoulder at the two o'clock point, precisely where the swell of breast tissue started to come up off her ribs. Not an ounce of fat was discernible on her body, nor was there a line apparent in her face. But inside, she was miserable.

"I've always taken really good care of myself. Look, it's like baby skin," she said, holding out an arm glistening like a peeled peach. She was proud of having a DNA glow—all from a diet of boneless, skinless sardines she read about in the Seventies in *Cosmopolitan.*

So what was she doing in an osteoporosis clinic, with all those brittle women suffering from low bone mass who have smoked and been slothful about exercise? Well, Sand's own mother had broken her pelvis. But we're not going to be like our mothers, are we? Sand belongs to the first generation of the new fifties woman. She has exercised almost every day of her life. "So I figured I'd postpone all of this. It wouldn't even get to me. The first time I even thought about it was in an exercise class at Sportsclub-L.A. Dyan Cannon, Teri Garr, Magic Johnson, they all go there—it's the stars' gym. I see the tushies of everyone. There's hardly a woman there who has her own breasts. And you can be sure none of *them* ever had menopause."

She was near the end of class, on the floor, grinding the old lower abs into the ground with leg lifts, when she started to perspire profusely. She thought, *What a great teacher!* "But later in the afternoon I was in Gelsons—it's like one of the best supermarkets in L.A.—and I started to have that feeling again. Oh-oh, maybe it wasn't just the great instructor." Dorian Gray time! *You're going to catch me being old.*

Sand was a dental hygienist: "I cleaned the teeth of the stars." She also had a new man in her life, a husband-to-be. She was in her psychiatrist's office when another hot flash hit, so she asked him about it. "If I were you," he said, "I would never mention menopause to this man." She followed the shrink's advice and hid her little secret from the man she married, which wasn't easy once she started having the night sweats.

Just beyond REM sleep—*bolt!*—she'd pop up like burnt toast. A minute later the sweating would start from every pore. Swiftly and silently she'd slip out from under the sheets and take a cold sponge bath, but sometimes her husband would awake and grumble, "Hey, it's wet in here! Jesuschrise, whatsammatta with these *sheets?*"

"I'm just having a little anxiety," she'd say, rubbing his head.

"But then around the same time your vagina starts to get dry. Also, I felt no desire." Now she was talking about a flagging of libido as the estrogen level drops and the tissues of the vaginal wall becomes thinner and drier. "Imagine discussing *that* with your mate," said Sand. "Unless you have a really decent guy, talking to him about menopause is like taking hemlock."

So Sand slid into bed as if she still belonged to a world of perfectly matched D-cup mango breasts and record arousal times, convinced that all she needed to do to enter the state of fifty-year-old erotica was "the mere act of holding a position for a count of thirty or forty seconds." She was thinking, *I'll be a menopause centerfold. I have this glistening body, right?* At the peak of a hot flash—*you want a hot woman? This is a hot woman.* Her new husband maneuvered her into position. And then, *it hurt.*

"It's hard to decide which came first, not wanting to have sex, or not wanting it because it hurt," said Sand.

Finally she sat her husband down and told him the facts of life. "I'm going through my Change of Life." Blank look. "I'm going through menopause." Her husband gave her a new name: My Change-of-Life Beauty Queen. She winced; it was a kiss with a kick.

The "Who Needs Men?" Argument

$\mathcal{F}$ay Weldon, the novelist known internationally for her wickedly wry chronicles of the battle between the sexes, observes in her novel, *Life Force,* ". . . when estrogen levels sink in a woman, it is safe for society to give her hormone replacement therapy, which keeps a female soft, sweet, and smiling, but antisocial to give the aging man testosterone injections, for if you do he runs round raping women and hitting other men on the head. What a bummer!" In the novel four women of a certain age are revisited by the same old lover, Leslie of the Magnificent Dong, who is sixty years old but still intent upon using his vital ten inches to revive infidelities of the past . . . "leaping, unstoppable, like electricity, from this one to that one, burning us up, making us old," as one of his menopausal targets describes the experience. But testosterone for women? The intriguing possibilities hadn't yet occurred to Weldon. One can't wait to see what her imagination might do with that new wrinkle.

I visited Weldon in the leafy Kentish Town section of London. A great blond Valkyrie of a woman, feet planted firmly in the earth of her tiny townhouse garden, she was waiting outside to welcome me. We threaded our way through her sun-splashed work parlor, past a grown son slumped in a beanbag sofa on the phone, and into a small solarium. All around were bunches of beautiful, blowsy late-summer roses, their petals splayed wide open, a rather apt simile for the attractive Earth Mother who sat before me.

In her mid-fifties, Weldon still sees sex as a necessary indulgence that both men and women need to survive. "I suppose, by and large, men have more opportunity to be sexually active as they grow older," she told me, "but I think women remain more sexually alive."

There is an important and poignant exception to this view. It's what Germaine Greer is trying to get at when she talks about having rejected hormone replacement. "When I used it myself, I didn't like that feeling of going back into the cycle," she said in an interview on CNN. She had already been postmenopausal for awhile, and having "glimpsed another place" beyond sexual desire, she "wanted to get back there."

If a woman no longer feels competitive or graceful in the guise of sexual huntress, she might well take the attitude, "Good riddance, who needs men?" The argument against hormone replacement then comes from an entirely new orientation: Life without sex can be more peaceful and allow one to get more done. And, in truth, it may make some women happier than continuing along in the same state of emotional frenzy—open to humiliation, rejection, anxiety, and misery as well as to the pleasures of sex. The woman's underlying fear here is that after a certain age, her face can't be saved, her body is going, and she probably can't find a suitable lover.

This may explain in part why some women start replacing their hormones and then stop. While they were not circulating much of their own hormones, desire may have slowly ebbed. One doesn't really notice. But if it's restimulated by taking hormones, one realizes that there is always another level of sexual tension that runs along underneath, rendering one vulnerable to expectation and disappointment. Once it's back, and she is an older woman, her options are to satisfy it or to sustain an inconsolable longing. Throwing out the pills or patches, then, may have less to do with sore breasts or feeling puffy than the need to take herself out of play. Otherwise, she opens herself to hurt again. It's not easy to put one's finger on it, because the vulnerability is not just to sexual longing. It is opening oneself again to the possibility of being in love.

Sex and the Single Woman of a Certain Age

By and large, the women who have a problem with sexuality in middle life are old married women, like me," believes Janine O'Leary Cobb, editor of *A Friend Indeed,* the Canadian menopause newsletter. "Many of us feel we had great sex when we were younger, and we don't mind if we have less now." But Cobb gets letters from women fifty and fifty-two who have taken new, younger lovers. "They're hot to trot and having a lovely time; sex was never so good."

Thus is born a new Old Wives' Tale, in which women pass the word about the tonic effect of a Change-of-Life Lover. The head of a department at a prestigious university was in her mid-forties when she first heard about it from a woman in her mid-fifties. The older woman told her to look forward to menopause: Pregnancy worries went out the window, and she'd had an affair of *grande passion* at that time—starting at forty-nine.

"I was stunned," recalls the younger woman. She is petite and had always prided herself on being taken for younger than she was, but the habit of marriage to a man she had known for several decades had made a buried treasure of her erotic self. Then, suddenly, she found herself swept up in an affair. When? She smacks her forehead with the insight: "It's only now I recognize *I* was the same age! Maybe I thought, *Forty-nine—last chance.*"

Gloria Steinem, known not only as the inspiration of the American feminist movement but as one of the most sexually animated women of her time, was delightfully frank when I asked her what a fulfilling sex life means to her now, having passed fifty.

"I am about to say a series of things that if I had heard them ten years ago, I wouldn't have believed them." She laughed. "All the readers of this should brace themselves—just have faith that it may be true for them, too." She laughed again. "Sex and sensuality—going to bed for two entire days and sending out for Chinese food—was such an important part of my life, and it just isn't anymore. It's still there, but it's less important. I don't know how much of it is hormonal and how much is outgrowing it."

Her face seemed more relaxed. She lay back against her sofa cushions, this peripatetic woman who had scarcely spent more than a few days at a time in her own apartment in the past twenty years, and she looked, at last, at home. "It doesn't really matter whether sex goes or doesn't go," she summed up. "What matters is that the older woman can choose whether it goes or not."

Carmen Callil, a high-powered London book publisher, chuckles when she thinks back on the "revolting promiscuity" that she and her generation of the feminist vanguard engaged in during the Sixties and Seventies. "I was obsessed with sex then," she admits. "But when you're younger, sex is about other things, too—

adventure, boldness, identity." Like Steinem, she never married. "There's no doubt about it, I'm not as interested in sex as I used to be." Sex has taken a place in her postmenopausal life comparable to television. Nice, but if she has something better to do, not now.

In championing the embrace of "manlessness," Germaine Greer claims that half the women of menopausal age will be without a man in their bed anyway. This is a greatly exaggerated estimate. In the U.S. March 1990 National Census, the percentage of forty-five to fifty-four-year-old women who were single, widowed, divorced, or married with a spouse absent totalled one quarter of their age group.

Happily married women or those who continue to enjoy having men in their lives cannot buy into militant celibacy. Newswoman Eve Pollard says, "For those of us who are trying to juggle nine lives, including a long-term relationship with a man, the idea that because you stop menstruating, you should pack it all in, is nonsensical. I would be the first one to say, if you're not terribly happy with this boring man, and don't want to wash his socks, why wait till you have the menopause? Get out before. Who knows who you might meet?"

In sum, women who are bothered by having their sexual aliveness revived on hormones may find in physical symptoms the excuse to withdraw. The very possibility of being open again to hurt causes so many women, discarded or ignored by men, to say, "Why bother?" But in not bothering to revive their sexual desire, they may ignore caring for their bodies and mental well-being.

Testosterone
for Women

❧

"*D*o I have to accept this?" is a question increasingly being asked by dynamic women in their fifties who are at the peak of their careers but alarmed to find their sexual pilot light abruptly lowered. Treatment with very small amounts of testosterone—always combined with estrogen—is becoming more commonplace.

Due to a drop in estrogen, many mid-life women experience sexual discomfort and dysfunction such as vaginal dryness and atrophy of the genitals. "Estrogen deficiency really does have a major impact on sexual functioning as it relates to genital health," says Sheryl Kingsberg, a clinical psychologist and assistant professor at Case Western Reserve School of Medicine. "However, it has little impact on sexual drive. For drive we look to androgens—a decline in testosterone during menopause is associated with a decrease in sexual drive in women. There are some strong arguments in favor of androgen replacement."

Postmenopausal women who come into the McGill University menopause clinic in Montreal, Canada, often say, "The kids are gone, my husband and I like each other, we do lots more things together now. But I find I'm simply not interested in sex. Maybe I don't really love him." Certain women notice the falloff in desire quite suddenly, reports Barbara Sherwin, associate professor of psychology in the university's obstetrics-gynecology department and codirector of the clinic. "When I can date it to the onset of menopause or several years thereafter, or to surgical menopause, in women who didn't have that complaint before, we suspect what they are missing is testosterone."

Scientific measurements have established that the testosterone level goes down by about one-third in the average postmenopausal woman who still has her ovaries. If her ovaries are removed, the fall is twice as great. The figures come from an acknowledged expert in hormone measurement, Dr. Howard Judd.

"Every woman has been told, 'Don't worry, your adrenals take over,' but the point is, the adrenals don't take over," insists Dr. Lila Nachtigall of NYU. The adrenal glands make about two-thirds of the testosterone circulating in the body of young women. But from the age of thirty on, a woman's adrenal glands slow down. Preliminary studies by Dr. Nachtigall show that after the ovaries are removed or shut down in postmenopause, the adrenal glands produce very little testosterone. What they do make is mostly in fat tissue of the body. "So if the woman is thin, she also has less testosterone," notes Dr. Sherwin.

In a small proportion of women the ovaries go on overtime—producing more testosterone than even during their reproductive life. These are the women who notice an increased sex drive; some will develop an enlarged clitoris. They may also see some hair appearing on their upper lips or chin; or a slight recession of hair at the temples; or a deepening voice. A woman who wonders about her testosterone level can have it measured from a blood sample; good norms exist. But she would have to ask for it.

Adding a testosterone preparation to estrogen replacement improves well-being and energy levels, especially in surgically menopausal women. It also revives sex drive and, often, cognitive functioning. More important, while estrogen alone stops additional bone loss, testosterone preparations help to rebuild depleted bone. Physicians and scientists are trying to determine if testosterone is necessary to maintain female muscle mass and bone density into old age. They are divided over the wisdom of giving postmenopausal women small doses of testosterone along with the estrogen replacement therapy they may receive. Although recent evidence is mixed, doctors worry that testosterone may negatively affect cholesterol, thus raising the risk of heart disease.

Dr. Barbara Sherwin, who has been conducting research on estrogen-testosterone combinations for fifteen years, has had women on this combination of drugs, by injection, for up to twenty years with good results. She cautions that with a full dose of testosterone about 20 percent developed some facial hair. When she cut the dose in half, less than 5 percent of women had any side effects. When given by injection, testosterone had no effect on HDL and LDL cholesterol levels. But it had a powerful effect on restoring libido and well-being in women who have had hysterectomies and who produce very little of their own testosterone.

Testing for testosterone levels is expensive (around $100) and usually unnecessary. Even if results show a woman has "normal" levels of the hormone, those levels may be insufficient in her particular case. "For those postmenopausal women who find themselves having difficulty with arousal and reaching orgasm," says Dr. Estelle Ramey, "a small amount of testosterone can make a big difference."

Vaginal Estrogen

*W*omen who have had breast cancer are now, for the first time, able to use small doses of vaginal estrogen to make sex possible. For women who have frequent urinary infections and trouble controlling frequency, and whose lack of estrogen causes so much dryness and thinning of the vaginal tissues that it makes sex very painful, the addition of even a small amount of vaginal estrogen can add enormously to the quality of their lives. Since it is almost completely absorbed, locally, most breast cancer specialists are comfortable with this treatment.

When I checked back with Gayle Sand, she had been told by a female doctor about a very low dose of Premarin used vaginally as a medication to maintain lubrication and keep tissue from thinning in the vaginal walls. "The effects were great," she exclaimed. "I have a normal sex life again." But she had also started a campaign to end the taboo. She'll speak up in an elevator: "Is it warm in here, or am I having a hot flash?" When the occupants gasp, giggle, then cluck, *"You,* you're too young for that," Sand sings back, "No, I'm not. I'm menopausal."

Over-the-counter preparations can restore moisture to the tissues of the vagina *without* the use of hormones. Gloria Bachmann, professor and chief of obstetrics and gynecology at the University of Medicine and Dentistry of New Jersey, along with Morris Notelovitz of the Women's Medical Center in Gainesville, Florida, conducted a one-year study demonstrating that Replens significantly increased vaginal health and quality of life in women suffering from vaginal dryness. The product works best when used on a continuous basis, rather than just prior to intercourse.

Educating
Your Man

❧

$\mathscr{M}$ost men go all twitchy when mention is made of anything to do with female reproductive organs or processes. They don't want to hear about your visit to the gynecologist, and they'll do *anything* to get out of making a run to the 7-Eleven to pick up tampons. There seems to be a hangover from primitive thinking that presupposes a woman is unclean when she is in cycle. And if she has "female troubles," the last person she can count on for a supportive ear may be her man. Those deep inner spaces are supposed to be only for pleasuring; they are not meant to have clinical names or flesh-and-blood malfunctions.

Patriarchal and primitive societies have done their part in prescribing the menstrual taboo. Just as they have fostered a division of women into two dimensions—good little ovulating wife who is the passive receptacle, and the scarlet woman or witch, who is active, sexually dynamic, and terrifying—men in traditional cultures have isolated the menstruating

woman as "unclean," "polluting," and "dangerous."
One would logically think that the woman who is
finished with the fearsome business of monthly bleeding would become better accepted, and in some
traditional cultures she is. But there is a new, subjective fear, and not just in primitive societies.

Middle-aged men, as they themselves begin to slow
down, have a good deal of fear and envy of the
physical, mental, sexual, and spiritual energies of
fully evolved women—women who are beyond being
objects defined by the male gaze and now fully
conscious keepers of their own bodies. That fear is
projected back onto women, causing us to wonder if
we really are over the hill when we no longer have
value primarily as erotic objects and reliable breeders.

In fact, married men are more apprehensive about
the effects of menopause on their life satisfaction than
women themselves. In a 1991 Gallup poll commis-
sioned by Ciba-Geigy, makers of the Estraderm
patch, one in four of the seven-hundred women aged
forty to sixty expressed concern about menopause,
but two thirds of the middle-aged husbands were
bothered about it. Only a third of the women were
satisfied with their husband's knowledge about the
Change of Life, and with good reason. Two thirds of
the husbands of premenopausal women expressed
fears that their sex lives would be compromised by
having a wife in menopause. A majority of the men
married to women in the transition focused on the
emotional impact on their wives, saying they mani-
fested anxiety, irritability, and mood swings. Fewer
than half the men took any notice of physical problems that underlay these emotional reactions, despite
the fact that the overwhelming majority of the women

in menopause reported struggling with hot flashes, night sweats, and difficulty sleeping.

A gynecological nurse at New York Hospital is struck by how men shun their wives when they come into the hospital for a hysterectomy. "The absence of the husband when it's an issue of female sex organs is so common," says Tanya Resilard. "And if they do come to visit, they seem afraid to go to the bedside. They want to be totally separate."

"My husband was incredibly supportive when I had breast cancer, but he really doesn't want to acknowledge I'm in menopause," I was told by a gutsy entertainer. Her spouse is a few years younger than she. When she tries to talk to him about having problems with concentration, he ascribes it to something else—it's stress or money problems or maybe flu—anything but the Change of Life. "He is in major denial about it—why?"

If you are getting older, so is your man. You may represent the mirror of his own aging. Breast cancer a husband can't catch. But aging is sex-neutral. Another woman who felt constrained about admitting to her husband she was struggling with menopause finally realized why. She was the second wife and represented to the husband his own renaissance. "He once told me, 'I don't ever want to think of you as middle-aged.'"

"In certain parts of the South they make you feel really shameful," notes Effie Graham, who grew up in Blanch, North Carolina, and is now a nurse's aide at New York Hospital. "The men refuse to let you sleep in the same room, tell you you're supposed to go through it alone. They had a lot of religious beliefs about menopause. They always said the Lord would take care of it."

As much as possible, it helps not to project one's own fears on the man. In fact, a woman can tell him, there is much to recommend a woman nearing the end of her reproductive stage. With the passing of pregnancy fears, her lustier fantasies can be played out with a refreshing lack of inhibitions. Best of all—and she must boast about this—she is soon to be free of the "blue meanies" that come with monthly cycles. The Gallup poll findings support this good news: Living through menopause puts far less strain on marriages than the apprehensions would suggest. A nearly identical majority of the husbands and wives polled—70 percent—acknowledged that, in fact, the women's interest in sex had not decreased during or after menopause. And two out of five of the women presently in the transition or just past it say that their relationship with their husbands has improved since menopause.

Estrogen
and
Brainpower

$\mathscr{A}$t forty you can't read the numbers in the telephone book. At fifty you can't remember them. What's going on?

There is mounting evidence that estrogen has a critical impact on the activity of the human brain—in both women and men—throughout the life cycle. Despite the fact that women over forty have superior stores of experience on which to draw in making sound decisions, as their estrogen levels begin to decline, they often experience problems such as forgetfulness, anxiety, and short-term memory loss. Shame and fear have traditionally kept them silent. But doctors report more working women are complaining about memory lapses, concentration problems, or lack of focus.

"I'm just not firing on all eight cylinders," admitted the creative director of a major cosmetics company to New York menopause expert, Dr. Patricia Allen. "Right in the middle of discussing a project, I'll forget that the week before we decided to use certain colors." She is joined by legions of working women who are worried about performing on the job, especially in high-stress positions that demand snap recall. Some fear their careers will be compromised.

Leading researchers are now investigating how estrogen crosses the "blood-brain barrier" to affect basic cognitive skills. "There is not a cell in the brain that is not estrogen-sensitive directly," announced Dr. Frederick Naftolin, professor and chairman of obstetrics and gynecology at Yale University, at the 1997 meeting of the American College of Obstetrics and Gynecology. "Every experimental study published so far indicates a lifelong relationship between [sex] hormones and the brain."

Seven years ago, when I first wrote about the estrogen effect on the brainpower of menopausal women, it was such a sensitive subject that some pioneering researchers begged me not to quote them by name for fear of a feminist backlash. Now that boomer women are beginning to experience the phenomenon, it is harder to sweep under the carpet.

Dr. Bruce McEwen, a neuroendocrinologist at Rockefeller University, has made some breakthroughs in tracking estrogen's effect on mental functioning since our first interview in 1991. He has demonstrated that estrogen increases the number of connections between nerve cells in the hippocampus, a region of the brain that helps keep track of the events in one's daily life. "Things that depend on reasoning or prior information require other memory banks," explains Dr. McEwen. "But just keeping track of what you did this morning, that's your hippocampus."

Estrogen is also very important in regulating moods and emotions, particularly anxiety and depression.

The absence of estrogen has a powerful effect on synapses at certain sites in the brain, explains Dr. McEwen. At Rockefeller University he has observed brain chemistry changes in rats during the equivalent of menopause (after their ovaries were removed). "The number of synaptic connections actually decreases. If you administer estrogens, these synaptic connections are remade within a few days." He emphasizes that the subjective experience of cloudy thinking at times during menopause can be equated, for instance, to jet lag: "It's mostly transient and certainly reversible."

Until now, memory lapses, mood changes, and lack of focus have been considered part and parcel of menopause. Many older women assume it just comes along with the aging process. But members of a new generation who have grown to midlife exercising a high degree of control over their bodies—from birth control to fertility manipulation—are demanding to know what to do about it.

Has Anyone Seen My Memory?

~

*B*ecky Stanton, a forty-six-year-old nurse from Ohio, recalls her own frustration with these symptoms. "None of the doctors seemed to take my complaints of difficulty concentrating and memory loss seriously," she recounts. "Not until my husband told them he was really worried—I had always been so 'on-the-ball,' he said, and now I was so 'airheaded.' He was scared that something was very wrong with me."

Strong women rely on their brainpower—it's their hard drive. "When you turn off your computer without going through all the right steps, you corrupt the files," says New York marketing consultant Mona Monaghan. "It seems like losing estrogen corrupts some women's files. And the linkages are not obvious. It's not just one thing you're going to forget. It's bits and bytes being lost all over the place. That worries me."

In young, healthy women, estrogen is the hormone

that helps to maintain verbal memory. It follows that as women lose estrogen with aging—beginning in their forties—there is an impact on brainpower. In my ongoing research on the menopausal passage, I often hear complaints like those of a very smart best-selling author whom I happened to phone one day. "How are you?" I asked.

"I'm thinking slower—are you? I have tremendous trouble concentrating. I start to write and just wander. Am I getting stupid?"

All writers have days like this. But this woman, just past fifty, was usually so witty about life's pitfalls. "What I feel is panic," she said. "I tape every interview now, because I know I won't remember. And I'm so intent on remembering, I become extremely irritable. Because if somebody interrupts me while I'm trying to remember, then I'm frightened of losing it."

She wasn't kidding. "You feel less competitive, slow off the mark. I think the bottom line is," she said glumly, "I'm just plain dimmer."

Wait a minute, hadn't she been all smiles after having had a hysterectomy? "Oh, sure, I was just so glad to be finished with cysts and fibroids," she remembered. The surgeon told her they had saved one ovary, which should produce enough estrogen so she wouldn't need to take hormones. That was three years before.

"You might be suffering from estrogen deprivation," I said.

"You mean, I'm not stupid, I just need hormones?"

I told her story to Dr. Barbara Sherwin. After the age of forty-eight, she said, the writer's remaining ovary would be quickly withering away. Moreover, manipulation during surgery to remove the uterus often compromises the blood supply to the ovaries. Professor Sherwin said she would be shocked if the writer's estrogen level weren't in the postmenopausal range. And the impact on mental acuity can be quite noticeable.

Sure enough, when my writer friend went to a gynecologist for her first pelvic exam in four years, the doctor said, "Your vaginal walls are bone-dry." She was in a state of estrogen deprivation. The writer decided to try a course of hormone replacement therapy. A few months later she told me, "I feel infinitely better, more alert, more moist, more like my old self." Having overcome her initial resistance to hormone replacement therapy, she now believes she will likely live a longer, healthier life. "You get on a track—with regular reminders to get mammograms and Pap smears. If something does go wrong, you have an early warning system set up to catch it." More pertinent, the author went on to produce her most meticulously reported and best-written book.

Dr. Sherwin has been doing studies for more than a decade on several hundred women in all stages of life. They are given standardized neuropsychological tests when they are estrogen-rich and when they are estrogen-deprived. The results are clear, says Dr. Sherwin. "Estrogen helps maintain verbal memory and it enhances a woman's capacity for new learning."

The working women who walk into Dr. Sherwin's menopause clinic often report, "Something has happened to my memory." They misplace things. It's harder to remember a new phone number, though they always remember the old ones. "People start getting methodical. They don't just put their glasses down on the kitchen counter; they put them down in a specific spot," notes Dr. Sherwin. Though this hormone-linked strain on short-term memory is quantifiable, most women are not seriously impaired in their daily functioning.

For a long while Dr. McEwen and Dr. Sherwin were lonely laborers in a field few scientists wanted to touch. All of a sudden there is an explosion of data showing that estrogen has a potent effect on keeping the brain tuned up, the sloughs of despondency at bay, and the specter of Alzheimer's disease at a safe distance.

Men, too, face a challenge to their mental vitality, as well as their virility, usually beginning in their fifties or sixties. This might be called the "male middle-life pause"—or MANopause—a five-to-twelve year period during which men go through hormonal fluctuations coupled with accelerated physical and psychological changes. Common symptoms of MANopause are irritability, a feeling of sluggishness, and mild to moderate mood swings. Memory and concentration may be affected in men, too, but the most fearsome symptom for men is a slump in sexual drive or intermittent failure to perform sexually. Dr. Tom Lue, an internationally renowned researcher and professor of the Department of Urology at the University of California at San Francisco, notes that almost all parts of the male body and metabolism slow down during the mid-fifties to the late sixties—an accelerated slide—

before they stabilize and a normal rate of attrition begins.

Among women, the few studies that show estrogen loss has a detrimental effect on mental functioning have been done on those who have had hysterectomies where the hormonal drop is sudden and acute. For naturally menopausal women, the effect may be a little fuzzy thinking in the early years of the Change. "When I was in my early fifties, it was impossible for me to look up in an index and hold three different page numbers in my head," chuckles Canadian newsletter editor Janine O'Leary Cobb. A few years later, new numbers and facts began again to stick to the coils of her memory. "Most of us do recover."

Given the new data, the link between estrogen and brainpower is beginning to be openly discussed. By 1997, when psychologist Claire Warga wrote a story in *New York* magazine asking "Can Estrogen Make You Smart?" she was able to quote Patricia Ireland, president of the National Organization for Women, bravely admitting to some of her own cognitive lapses before she started hormone replacement therapy. "All of us who are honest in our philosophy and our politics have to be willing to look at what the studies are showing," says Ireland.

Recent studies of estrogen's benefits on the brain have come to several intriguing conclusions:

- Estrogen may act as an antioxidant and anti-inflammatory agent that can inhibit age-related deterioration of brain cells.

- Estrogen elevates mood and may protect against depressive illness.

- Estrogen may reduce the risk of Alzheimer's disease by more than 50 percent.*

Thus, estrogen has recently been posited as a woman's best defense against organic brain disease in later life. Although women on average live longer than men, the burden of Alzheimer's disease falls more heavily on women than men. Based on studies at the University of Southern California, Dr. Victor Henderson proposes that plummeting levels of circulating estrogens after menopause increase a woman's risk of this disorder and, conversely, that estrogen replacement therapy may lower the risk for dementia due to Alzheimer's disease.

Some women say their memory becomes more acute than ever after they start taking estrogen. The hormone also spurs the production of an important enzyme in the brain that helps the connections between brain cells to flourish, making it quicker and easier for messages to leap from one neuron to the next. The inside of a robust, estrogenized brain might look more like the dense telephone wiring in an urban telephone terminal box, while the brain of an older, estrogen-deprived woman or man might look more like the sparse wiring of a rural telephone substation.

The results are most dramatic in healthy, functioning women who are tested just before they have a

---

* One study derived from the Baltimore Longitudinal Study of Aging indicated that those who had taken estrogen had a 54 percent lower risk of Alzheimer's disease than those who had never used the hormone. Another study, conducted by researchers at Columbia University, followed 1,124 women in New York City and showed that taking estrogen for a year or longer reduced the risk of Alzheimer's disease by 87 percent.

hysterectomy in which their ovaries are removed.
After the operation, their scores on tests of verbal
memory and retention of new material decrease significantly. But Dr. Sherwin is quick to point out that
they could still perform reasonably in their jobs and
manage their lives. However, those who were given
estrogen therapy postoperatively performed compara-
tively better. All the women she has tested decided to
take hormone replacement once the trials were completed.

But what about the years after menopause?

Growing and Regenerating Brain

✍

$\mathcal{O}$nce past menopause, many of today's women find themselves blazing with renewed energy and raring to go. They are returning to school, starting their own businesses, mounting causes, doing radio talk shows, running for public office, and needing to exercise their gray matter rather than letting it turn to pudding.

The prevailing view in the 1960s was that the human brain goes through a fixed number of cell divisions and then the cells die. Dr. Caleb Finch, also at USC and a pioneer in the study of sex hormones in the aging process, corrects that view: "It is apparent that there is no such rigid programming to the human life span."

Here is the really good news: Our most basic fears about mental decline with aging are challenged by recent research. Brain cells do not automatically die off as we age in one-hundred-thousand cell lots, as was erroneously reported. There is some cell death, but mostly brain cells shrink or grow dormant in old age, particularly from lack of stimulation and challenge.

Dr. Marion Diamond, an eminent neuroscientist, is former director of the Lawrence Hall of Science at the University of California, Berkeley, and is still actively teaching, researching and mentoring. At age seventy, she has no plans to retire. Why? "Because of what we have learned from our rats," says Dr. Diamond, an attractive statuesque blond woman with a mind like a whiplash. "Just because we have wrinkled faces doesn't mean that the brain doesn't have potential." After forty years of experimentation and analysis, Dr. Diamond can give this assurance:

"There is no significant loss of brain cells—in the healthy brains of people who are living normal, healthy lives—all the way up through old age."

The difference between "healthy brains" and dimming bulbs depends to a great extent on the amount of daily mental stimulation. Animals or people placed in impoverished environments (without toys or friends) show degeneration in brain cells. But rats— or people in middle or late age—when placed in enriched environments with lots of objects to work or play with and lots of friends to socialize with, show enhancement in their brain cells. It appears that if people seek out vigorous mental stimulation on a daily basis—doing computations or crossword puzzles, learning a new computer program, playing furious contract bridge—even an older, developed brain can grow, sprouting new neural foliage and making new connections.

Where to Find Your Memory

*N*ormal aging often entails mental slowing, changes in visual/spatial orientation, and some memory loss. But you can maintain what you have, ward off losses, and possibly regain some of what you lost—even without taking hormones. The following are natural brainpower boosters:

• ANTIOXIDANTS

All aging is caused by oxidative damage to tissues. You can slow the process considerably by adding a comprehensive antioxidant formula to your daily diet including beta carotene, selenium, zinc, vitamins C, E, and the B complex—especially niacin and vitamins B-1, B-3, B-5, and B-6, along with folic acid.

• NUTRITIONAL SUPPLEMENTS

A new class of chemical-free natural supplements derived from plant and vegetable sources are on the market. Traditionally prescribed to patients suffering from early Alzheimer's disease, supplements like phosphatidylserine (derived from soy) are increasingly being used by complementary physicians to treat memory loss and promote cognitive functioning in postmenopausal women.

• MOVEMENT LEARNING

Playing a new sport, fixing an appliance, or keeping track of steps in an aerobics class will exercise the mind as well as the body. Learning new patterns and sequences of movement tones your brain and boosts overall function in both short- and long-term memory.

• CONTENT LEARNING

Memorize a Shakespearean sonnet, take a course in French cooking or Greek Mythology at your local college, read a section of the paper you usually skip. Such activities are the equivalent of pumping the iron in your mind. Most importantly, find something that you feel passionate about and concentrate on learning all you can about it.

• SOCIAL LEARNING

Studies have shown that older people with close partners reinforce their own memories through their daily dialogue, which enhances memory retention. Social interaction will help you branch out and reinforce your neural pathways *and* relationships. So get out and socialize! Join the church choir, organize museum outings with a group of friends. If you're retired, volunteer for a charity, a political campaign or a nonprofit organization.

The
Menopause
Gateway

$\mathcal{S}$ome women have genetic good fortune. Even after entering menopause, they continue to make enough female hormone precursors in their adrenal glands, and to make enough estrogen from these precursors in their fat deposits, so that they do not experience any symptoms or, at most, only temporary hot flashes. This pause is a marker event in their lives, but it does not take on the physical or psychological freight of a major event.

"They are thrilled not to have to deal with the menstrual cycle anymore, and some of them seem to maintain their bone levels very well," observes Theresa Galsworthy, the nurse-clinician who directs the Osteoporosis Center at the Hospital for Special Surgery in New York. Broad-scale figures on the proportion of women who fall into this fortunate group are probably impossible to come by, but activity at the Osteoporosis Center offers a clue. "During the course of the week about fifteen patients come to me to have their bone density measured because they're fairly newly postmenopausal. Maybe two or three of the fifteen have absolutely no symptoms," says Galsworthy. These women are usually on the older side of the norm when they experience the Change, fifty-one or fifty-two.

Women who deal with menopause by denying it entirely become easy to pick out. They are the ones you see eating a lettuce leaf and glass of seltzer for lunch, their hair color slightly lurid, their time more and more taken up with becoming skillful makeup artists or searching for the right cosmetic surgeon. The results may be admirable, and mask the years, but sooner or later time and nature will catch up with us all.

Strenuous dieting at this age, for instance, is the worst way to preserve one's long-term health and grace. Estrogen is stored in the body's fat cells. Some researchers differentiate between the Thin Woman's Menopause and the Plump Woman's Menopause, the latter usually being far less symptomatic. "In populations where women don't get carried away with wearing a size six dress when they're fifty-five, and they still do regular exercise and they're not smoking, bone fractures are not much of a problem," says Dr. Elizabeth L. Barrett-Connor, a top epidemiologist at the University of California, San Diego.

At the opposite extreme are women who allow themselves to become "victims" of menopause, using this time of life as an excuse to become inactive, go to fat, beg off sex, and sulk, often leading them to depression and the door of menopause clinics. These are the middle-aged women who perpetuate the stereotype of the menopausal woman as synonymous with "mean old bitch."

The professional women I have studied are accustomed to considerable control over their environment, and they have worked hard to achieve it. They pride themselves on being fiercely organized and prepared for just about any crisis. These mid-forties dynamos can fax a dinner menu to a caterer, sell a stock, talk supportively to a spouse over a portable phone without missing a step, and remember to take their aerobics shoes to the office along with their satin slingbacks so they'll be able to exercise before appearing glamorous at the AIDS benefit. But they cannot control when they break out in a hot flash or when they bleed.

The meanest loss of menopause, for them, is the sudden loss of control. Among high-performing professionals, puzzlement often develops into panic followed by outrage. That was the route traveled by Meredith, a mother of two and model business leader in her middle-American community, who had stopped counting birthdays at thirty-eight. That was the year she went into business and consciously knew she looked terrific and felt the same way.

She started having mysterious migraines at forty-two. They grew more frequent. Over the next ten years she traipsed around to one gynecologist after another, all of whom posited psychological causes— i.e., "Type A's are often migrainous." At age fifty Meredith was the one to insist upon a blood test that would measure her hormones. She had zero estrogen and zero progesterone. Now completely frustrated, she saw a TV commercial for a menopause clinic in

Cleveland, Ohio. She flew there to have a bone densitometer test, which revealed she had 10 percent less bone mass than the norm for women her age. Not one doctor up to then had mentioned her bones in connection with menopause or brought up the risk of osteoporosis.

"I feel like I dropped a percentage point of bone mass in each one of those doctor's offices," Meredith says ruefully. She also wonders, with good reason, if the migraines were the result of estrogen depletion over the past ten years.

I recognized her immediately when we first met. It was the walk, perhaps. Her long legs took the sidewalk one full paving stone at a time, high heels notwithstanding. She was good-looking, still blond and pink-complexioned, the parentheses at either side of her mouth lending animation to her face. Her friends had described her as "dynamic, tough, successful, and doesn't take no for an answer." Her real estate company will do 55 million dollars of business this year, and her mortgage banking company will do 80 million.

"You'd think I could manage my period, right?" Meredith wisecracked. Fifty—the number itself—held no menace for her, she said, although it came out that the year Meredith turned fifty, her mother died of breast cancer. It was her first personal experience with death, immediately followed by the onset of menopause. "And something happened to me, I don't know what, I became a little nutsy about flying in an airplane. I began to feel a foreshortening of time." Meredith said she was too busy to figure it out.

"I've been obsessed," she says. "Menopause is the only thing that's made me feel I had an age. Because I can't get rid of it. I hate it, big time."

During a group interview, Meredith held up the computerized cost-benefits chart she had designed to analyze whether or not to take hormone replacement therapy. The impressive-looking graph was all the more infuriating to her because there was no bottom line. "So what do I go for? Cancer, osteoporosis, or heart disease?"

For her, menopause represents her lack of control over mortality. Many of us don't have to face up to mortality until our mothers die. The loss of that unconditional love leaves no cushion between ourselves and the outrages of life, no grip against a suddenly perceived slippage on "the downward path" toward one's own inevitable "dusty death." Control becomes magnified in importance. In reaction, Meredith developed her new phobia about airplanes, where as a passenger she could exercise no control. Still, she had pushed away any conscious recognition of her aging until the physical insults of menopause finally made it impossible to remain, even in her own mind, thirty-eight.

Now, faced with making a medical decision about her life that involves the breast cancer issue, with the loss of her mother not yet mourned, Meredith is in a constant state of conflict. She longs to escape from her own success: "Being a mentor is a burden. I feel like I'm not creating anything new." She resents her husband's assumption that he will take early retirement. " 'What about me?' I feel like saying. 'When can I retire?' " She is unconsciously afraid that she will follow her mother before she has had time to live fully. All these fears and frustrations have been focused on the secondary issue of menopause. And they come out as anger.

To make matters more frustrating, the cost-benefit analysis on how to treat menopause resists adding up to any clear, rational, risk-free answer. Why? Because we don't have enough data. And because everything has a price. A well-informed, affluent woman like Meredith might well decide, "Well, hell, if I know hormones are going to protect my heart, my mind, and my bones, I guess I can monitor my breasts with mammography and my uterus with ultrasound, and see how it goes." Or she may prefer to try to manage the whole process naturally.

Partnering Yourself Through a Natural Menopause

~

*M*any women resist medicalizing a natural event such as the Change. Others, like Serafina Corsello, have little choice.

"I had a wonderful defense, called denial," admits Dr. Corsello, an elegant European woman who practices nutritional medicine at the Corsello Center on Manhattan's West Side. She was simply never going to have all those unseemly symptoms other women report, poor things. Blessed with high energy and an insatiable desire for learning beyond dogma, Corsello completed a medical internship and residency in New York. Throughout her thirties she juggled a classical medical practice with being a single mother. But in her early forties she became disenchanted with mainstream medicine. The outcome of her midlife crisis was a commitment to educate herself in complementary medicine—vitamin therapy and other natural procedures—realizing that it meant she would have to study every day for the rest of her life.

"Will I be able to keep up this level of performance?" she worried as she plunged into self-education, taking on new financial burdens as well as committing to a second marriage. But at fifty she found she still had fantastic energy, having always been able to hit the pillow and sleep within two seconds.

"At fifty-two all of a sudden I'd hit the pillow, and hit the pillow—at two in the morning I'd still be hitting the pillow. This was the first sign; it was devastating."

It took Dr. Corsello no time to get an estrogen patch and congratulate herself on reregulating her sleep. She was herself again for the next two years. "One day I woke up and felt an ominous mass in my breast." The large cyst made her suddenly aware of the history of cancer in her family. She looked at her lovely little patch and synthetic progesterone pills and said, *"Adieu, chérie."*

She doctored herself with Chinese herbs, indulged in a massage once a week, and concentrated on creating a new aesthetic in her life. She surrounds herself with classical music; even in her office it is constantly in the background, soothing her. Since she loathes exercise but loves dancing, Dr. Corsello built in her own unique daily stress-reducing activity. She shuts the bedroom door while she watches a tape of the *NewsHour* and throws herself into high-paced disco dancing, all by herself.

Today at age sixty-five, elegant and vivacious, Serafina Corsello has taken a ten-year lease on her office in Manhattan—a powerful statement of her belief that "I'm not only in my prime now, but I'm still on my way up." Like many professional women, she is operating under a different time line from her male peers. Her career development was delayed by single motherhood and slowed slightly by menopause. "I couldn't stop at sixty because I had hardly begun," she says enthusiastically. But there is nothing stopping her now. She works every day, and on weekends she studies and writes. "The constant intellectual stimulation allows my mind and body to remain attuned. I keep on improving," she says.

The greatest reward of sixty-plus years of experience, she finds, is mental efficiency. She can actually sense her right and left brains, working in synchrony. And with this wide spectrum of intellectual capacity, she says, "We can zoom in to get the whole picture." She now expresses her ideas on health care *without fear* of offending the male medical establishment. She no longer labors under the younger woman's apprehensions—'What if I'm not right?" or, "Oh, my God, will they be offended?"

"Do you know how much energy this saves?" she says, twinkling. "I used to go into preambles—'you know' and 'on the other hand'—but I've cut fifty percent of that—it's freedom!" As she says now, "If I'm not right, well, I'm not right. This attitude allows you to shortcut all the tangents you had to go through as a young woman—because no longer being a sexual object, you're no longer trying to *please* anybody. At this point what is important to me is elegance. And elegance has nothing to do with sex." The greatest change she has noticed is the aesthetic confidence she has developed as an older woman.

Dr. Corsello has explored most of the herbal preparations popularly used to ease menopausal symptoms. She finds the most effective to be dong quai, a Chinese herbal remedy. "If I'm under stress, bingo, I take thirty or forty little drops and find miraculous relief." She suggests a woman ask a Chinese herbalist to make up a mixture to suppress hot flashes.

"I don't believe in using only one thing, I believe in the synergy between herbs," says Dr. Corsello. She has developed a Meno-Pak that contains all the herbs and supplements she would recommend.

Dr. Denning Cai, a highly experienced Chinese medicine doctor in Tarzana, California, sees many high-profile women in the Los Angeles area who are so terrified of menopause, they actually bring it on themselves earlier.

"People with an aggressive personality—women who try so hard to reach something, who feel 'I have to,' and who push themselves hard all the time—put the body under higher stress," Dr. Cai observes, "and this can bring on the menopause sooner." If she works with such women early enough to rebalance and calm their bodies, sometimes the menopause is delayed.

The theory in Chinese medicine is that energy in the kidneys begins to decline for women around the age of forty-nine, and so it was written in the ancient Chinese texts. Today, a practitioner would assess the individual woman and make up a mixture of herbs to revitalize her kidney function.

The Indian homeopathic tradition, as practiced by the world-renowned Shyam S. Singha, who has several clinics in London and one in Suffolk, is to treat menopause entirely through diet and homeopathic remedies. He finds the agnus castus herb particularly helpful in rebalancing estrogen and progesterone levels. Almonds, soaked overnight and peeled, are very rich in calcium. Some women report they obtain relief of hot flashes and sweats from acupuncture. Vitamin E is commonly used to relieve hot flashes. Primrose oil is another longstanding remedy. It contains gamma-linolenic acid, which helps mediate hormonal activity.

Women who frequent the health spa at Rancho La Puerta volunteered that acupuncture once a month has helped them with hot flashes and night sweats that disturb sleep as well as alleviating dry vagina.

The most helpful modifications you can make in your diet are:

1. Decrease fat intake

2. Increase calcium intake

3. Increase the tofu in your diet (but tofu is high in fat, so it has to be balanced out). You can make mayonnaise or salad dressing out of tofu or use it with yogurt as a vegetable dip.

4. Eat *yams*—a source of natural plant estrogen. Yams also have lots of beta carotene in them which is an antioxidant and will help support your immune system.

The best natural defense against osteoporosis is to keep the acidity of your blood in proper balance. If you don't, your body will, removing calcium from your bones to defend the pH balance in the blood. Blood acidity is caused, first and foremost, by chronic stress. Therefore, it is of the utmost importance for any woman over forty-five, faced with high-stress professional or personal demands, to commit herself to some restorative relaxation measure. It might be biofeedback, prayer, yoga, or routine meditation.

I find much wisdom in the ancient Hindu health system known as Ayurveda. The guiding principle is that any disorder can be prevented as long as balance is maintained, in the mind and spirit as well as in the body. Dr. Deepak Chopra, one of the first M.D.'s to introduce Ayurvedic theory and practice in the West, explains in his book, *Perfect Health:* "The mind exerts the deepest influence on the body, and freedom from sickness depends upon contacting our own awareness, bringing it into balance, and then extending that balance to the body. This state of balanced awareness, more than any kind of physical immunity, creates a higher state of health."

From modern science we know that the hypothalamus, or "the brain's brain," is responsible for balancing everything that goes on automatically in the body. Less than an ounce of gray matter in the forebrain must simultaneously balance the body's temperature, rate of metabolism, and sleep, along with its growth, hunger, thirst, blood chemistry, respiration, and many other functions. For optimum health to be maintained, coordination by the hypothalamus must be as precise as the movements of a conductor with a 150-piece orchestra.

During the perimenopause and early phase of menopause, even the brain's brain is often thrown off by the unpredictable changes in a woman's internal hormonal milieu. Try as it might, sending desperate signals to the pituitary gland to activate more estrogen, the hypothalamic regulator is confused when the ovaries don't respond as they did before. It can't do its usual conducting job. Hence, the body is often out of balance. Good health is harder to maintain.

Many women will develop allergies for the first time during the menopausal transition. If the state of imbalance is allowed to become too extreme, and the immune system is weakened, the disease process sets in. Everyone recognizes the sensations that signal an upcoming cold or flu, even though they are vague. Similarly, a menopausal woman whose body is seriously out of balance will feel "out of sorts," tired, cranky, and may complain of vague discomforts that are the body's premonition of disease.

Most doctors are baffled or impatient with such reports (if a woman even thinks her complaints serious enough to take to a doctor). Unless a woman takes herself seriously, and invests some time in learning about her vulnerabilities at this time of life, she may wind up in illness.

What can you do for yourself?

The single most important aid to continued health through the menopausal transition is proper rest. When you feel that you are pushing yourself too hard or racing, stop and rest if only for five minutes. Even better, learn how to meditate. The most restful rest, aside from a night's sleep, is the deep relaxation experienced during the state of meditation. According to Dr. Chopra, the common symptoms of the "worried well" in menopause—headache, insomnia, low-level anxiety or depression—benefit most from the act of meditation. One can emerge thoroughly settled and refreshed after only a few minutes of transcending.

Become serious about regular exercise. Find something you like to do; best if it requires making an appointment or a social date because then you'll have to keep to it. But you can also park at the end of the shopping mall and walk briskly with march music on your Walkman. This physical effort will support your bones, heart, lungs, as it pumps oxygen for clear thinking and endorphins for good feelings straight to your brain.

It is not wise to drink alcohol or too much coffee while you are trying to rebalance your body. Moreover, to minimize loss of mineral from bone it is vital to keep the acidity level in your blood as low as possible. Smoking, alcohol, and coffee also raise acid levels in the blood. Even a nightly glass of wine can wreak havoc with a hormonal system already out of balance. Carbonated sodas and beef, both of which have a high phosphorus content, are particularly dangerous for postmenopausal women, advises Dr. Corsello. She suggests a diet that emphasizes vegetables, complex carbohydrates, fiber, fish, and vegetable proteins such as tofu.

No natural remedies can be guaranteed effective, and none, of course, is approved by the FDA. Bear in mind that no pharmaceutical company stands to cash in on herbal remedies, since they are natural and can be sold over the counter. And since drug companies fund much of the medical research, it is not surprising that there is no serious money going into the study of Chinese medicine and its impact on menopause.

The pledge to have a "natural menopause," while politically correct, presents some contradictions. Is it "natural" to live for decades beyond fifty? And to want to feel in our seventies the way we do now?

This will be the first generation to get old routinely, and one way or another its women will have to provide some things that Mother Nature did not. None of the herbal remedies protects against bone loss. Janet Zand, a Chinese medical practitioner in Los Angeles, claims that herbs can diminish atrophy of the vagina. But as estrogen levels decline, the vaginal tissues become thinner and dryer. Gradually, over the decade of menopause, the vagina will shrink in both length and width. One female gynecologist drew me a picture of the normal estrogenized vagina of a woman in her thirties. It looked about five inches long and the width of two middle fingers.

"In many women of sixty who have taken no estrogen, I can hardly insert my pinkie," said the gynecologist. If a woman discontinues hormone-replacement, the process of atrophy will start again. Doctors recommend that older women keep up an active sex life because that will keep the vaginal walls elastic. But the common reason that women don't "use it" and eventually "lose it" is that making love becomes naturally painful when the vagina shrinks in size. Estrogen cream, as explained, and new over-the-counter preparations do counteract the discomfort.

The
Hidden Thieves

Active women often take pride in toughing it out: "I was too busy to notice menopause—I just sailed right through it" is their refrain. They may not be fully aware of the hidden thieves of menopause: osteoporosis, cognitive changes, and heart disease. This knowledge must be factored in before any of us can make an intelligent decision about how best to manage our own menopause.

Start up a conversation with any group of women where the ratio of blond to gray has tipped well over the fifty-fifty standoff, and there will be one woman who proclaims righteously, "Hormones. Not me! I want to stay healthy." Another will insist smugly, "I love my estrogen, I wouldn't give it up for anything!" And another will be totally ambivalent, able to be talked into either decision. Elizabeth Barrett-Connor, the University of California epidemiologist, observes that women break down into these three camps.

Most women have become phobic about breast

cancer, with some good reason. Their fear, however, leaves them vulnerable to a greater threat. At each group interview I asked the participants to guess what they were most likely to die from. The answers always startled me. Nine out of ten women will say cancer, most of them specifying breast cancer. A few will throw in the possibilities of airplane or auto crashes. Almost no one mentions the number one killer of women over fifty.

Heart disease.

The
Cheating Heart

❧

*A*lthough the risk of heart attack does not increase abruptly at the moment a woman reaches natural menopause, the rate of heart disease does rise sharply over the course of the decade after a woman reaches her fifties.

One in two postmenopausal women will develop heart disease. Two out of three women will die of it.

Coronary heart disease kills approximately 233,000 women annually. "Then why don't we read about women having heart attacks the way we do men?" someone will sensibly demand. Perhaps because doctors pay less attention to women's symptoms of heart disease and treat them less aggressively than they do men. As a result, women often develop more advanced heart disease and are more likely to have fatal heart attacks than men. Two new studies involving tens of thousands of patients have recently shown irrefutable evidence of sex differences in the way heart conditions are treated. The unawareness of the general public simply reflects the prevailing attitude in the medical fraternity that heart disease is a man's disease.

Here is a typical story I hear during interviews. Judy is a Dallas woman married to a CPA named Jack, who had a coronary at age fifty-two. Jack is virtually paralyzed by his fear of a recurrence; he is afraid even to work. He and Judy used to take an aerobics class together, but he gave it up, so Judy stopped exercising, too. Jack gave up repairing things around the house, so Judy began to do more, even when she felt "gas pains" or tingling in her left arm. Jack even gave up sex. The beta blocker he was told to take interfered with his potency, and he was so ashamed of a faltering erection that he stopped sleeping with Judy, stopped hugging her, even stopped holding hands in the movies.

Years went on. Jack retired early, so Judy had to go back to working full-time—a stressful job as a complaints manager at a discount store. She started smoking again and binge-eating during her breaks. She was having menopausal symptoms—fatigue, waves of the blues, migraines—but she didn't think she had time to go for a checkup.

She went with her husband to *his* doctor to hear what *he* should do to prevent another heart attack. But Judy didn't mention to Jack's cardiologist that she was having chest pains, or that her ankles were swelling, or that her father had died of a coronary at forty-seven. At that point, Judy was probably at greater risk for a sneak heart attack than her husband.

Like so many women, she was more concerned with meeting everyone else's needs than in paying attention to her own.

Heart disease is still thought of as a man's problem. The truth is, cardiovascular disease is the leading killer of women over fifty. A woman's chance of dying from heart disease is more than double that of dying *from cancer of any kind*. It takes *ten times* as many women's lives as breast cancer.

Yet even when a woman does complain of tightness in the chest or breathlessness in the middle of the night, many doctors take a wait-and-see approach. Judy had all the main risk factors for heart disease, which can be slow-growing in women. Women can get away with a lot of risk factors in their thirties and forties, but once menopause shuts down their natural estrogen protection, women begin to approach the same risk level for heart disease as men.

The Nurses' Health Study, the first long-term study of women's health, in which 120,000 women subjects (mostly white) have been followed for twenty-two years, found striking results on the heart disease front. After ten years, 48,000 of the postmenopausal subjects—who had no histories of cancer or heart disease when the study began—were evaluated. "Women who were taking estrogen, after menopause, had just half as many heart attacks and cardiovascular deaths as women who never used estrogen," reported Meir Stampfer, who led the study. An evaluation by Dr. Lee Goldman of Brigham and Women's Hospital in Boston concludes, "The benefits of estrogen outweigh the risks, substantially."

A clear picture of the "cumulative, absolute risks"

of the major causes of death for white women—between the ages of fifty and ninety-four—were spelled out in an editorial accompanying the Nurses' Health Study. There is a 31 percent absolute risk of dying of heart disease, a 2.8 percent risk of dying of breast cancer, a 2.8 percent risk of a hip fracture, and only a 0.7 percent risk of uterine cancer.

"Women lag behind men in heart disease by about five to seven years," says Dr. Trudy Bush. "It really starts hitting women in their late fifties and sixties." By age sixty-seven women are just as likely to have a heart attack as their husbands, but more likely to die from it.

Another recent important finding of the Nurses' Health Study confirms that a high intake of two B vitamins—folate (or folic acid) and B-6—cuts the risk of heart disease nearly in half, and is as important to a woman's cardiovascular health as quitting smoking, lowering high cholesterol and controlling blood pressure. Although the Recommended Daily Allowance, or RDA, is currently set at 180 micrograms for folic acid and 1.6 milligrams for B-6, women will achieve maximum cardiovascular benefits by doubling—even tripling—the RDA, said Eric Rimm, director of the study, in a recent *New York Times* article. Folic acid and vitamin B-6 can be found either in supplements or in foods such as orange juice, spinach and other leafy greens, whole grains, bananas, potatoes, chicken and fish.

The most significant predictor of heart disease is the HDL level. Bad cholesterol levels normally increase in women for some ten to fifteen years following the cessation of periods. Again, dangerous changes in cholesterol count or blood pressure do not announce themselves with obvious symptoms, not until there is a medical catastrophe. "If your HDL level is low, and your LDL level is relatively higher— even if you're walking around with a total cholesterol count of 200—you're going to be in trouble," says Dr. Estelle Ramey. Estrogen replacement therapy decreases LDL (bad) cholesterol levels by about 15 percent and raises the HDL (good) cholesterol levels by the same amount.

Estrogen also has a direct effect on the wall of the blood vessels. "Cholesterol uptake is the first change that occurs in the creation of the plaque that forms the basis for heart disease," explains Dr. Robert Lindsay. "Estrogen appears to block that effect, resulting in open vessels and good blood flow."

So there are multiple ways in which estrogen reduces heart disease risk more than any other known drug, including the new designer hormones. At last, after a half-century of conflicting data, former Surgeon General Dr. Bernadine Healy confirmed, "We can confidently assert that estrogen reduces key cardiovascular risk factors in women at a time when they become especially vulnerable to heart disease, namely, after fifty years of age."

If your primary goal is to lower your risk of heart disease, you may want to take hormone therapy indefinitely. But any benefit eventually costs. The Postmenopausal Estrogen/Progestin Intervention— or PEPI trial, as it is known—studied 875 women over a period of three years and confirmed the already impressive evidence from the Nurses' Health Study: Estrogen taken alone or taken with progesterone cuts the potential of heart disease among women in half. It also reduces by 50 percent their risk of dying from a heart attack.

But after ten or more years on HRT, the dramatic drop in death rates was reduced by 20 percent as the woman's risk of death from breast cancer rose. So it's a tricky trade-off. The new study showed that women with one or more risk factors for heart disease were likely to derive the greatest mortality benefit from hormone replacement.

What can a woman like Judy do besides take hormones to reduce her exposure to heart disease? There are three critical steps:

Number one: Judy should quit smoking. Cigarettes are the leading cause of heart disease in women.

Number two: Judy should cut down the animal fat and trans-fat in her diet. The ideal midlife diet for women is:

- Low in fat and dairy products
- High in phytoestrogens—a great source is soy milk
- High in vegetables and fruits, especially those containing vitamin E and folic acid
- High in fiber
- Small portions—four or five little "meal-lets" a day

Number three: Judy should start exercising again and build up to a consistent exercise regimen. Researchers in menopause agree with most physicians: the single best investment a woman can make in her health and well-being is exercise. A sedentary life is now recognized as a major risk factor for heart disease—almost as great as smoking. 12 percent of all deaths in the United States are now attributed to inactivity.

The simplest form of exercise—one that everyone can do all one's life—is walking. Walking doesn't mean strolling (window shopping doesn't count). It means at least thirty minutes of brisk, disciplined walking every day, at least five days a week. Walking at least two miles a day makes the heart muscle a more effective pump and will slow your heart rate as well. Plus, you get more oxygen to the brain, which enables you to think better!

Number Four: Judy should also make an effort to reduce stress. Acute stress sets off a rush of adrenaline and other hormones that cause the heart to beat faster and blood pressure to soar. Repeated episodes of adrenaline rush damage the blood vessel linings and build up cholesterol deposits in the walls of the arteries, which is highly detrimental to cardiovascular health.

But how to reduce the stresses of everyday life, which perversely accumulate as new communications technologies keep us "on" virtually all the time? It isn't enough to take the pressure off for a week's vacation now and then. We need to break stride and build short "retreats" into our daily routine. Making time for meditation or yoga every day—alternating with exercise—can lower blood pressure quite amazingly. These relaxation techniques slow the heart rate and decrease symptoms of anxiety, anger, and depression, and are excellent ways of managing stress.

Embezzled Bone

❧

*M*argie is very good at giving care to everyone else—her laundry-toting postadolescent kids and the battered women she works with at the community center in her college town. Still blond, though aware she is white at the roots, Margie will turn fifty this year. "Oh, shit, my number's up" was her reaction. Her doctor told her ten years ago she was a sitting duck for osteoporosis—the second major thief of menopause. Small-boned, she remembers her statuesque mother shrinking about seven inches to a mere five feet tall before she died. "I already know I have bone thinning," she admits.

Typically she resists addressing the issue because that would mean her good-bye to youth. "I'll take hormones when I get there."

"What's *there?*" her girlfriend challenged her.

"You know, old."

Old is too old to start protecting bones. By the time anybody can *see* osteoporosis, it's too late to reverse it. As you'll recall, we begin to lose bone after the age of thirty-five; the normal rate of loss is about one percent a year. "The window of accelerated bone loss—and the opportunity to protect against it—is in the five years after menopause," says Dr. David Zackson, endocrinologist and research director of Calcium Metabolism at New York Hospital-Cornell Medical School. That is, when a woman hits fifty, bone loss accelerates to about a percent and a half each year for the next five to ten years, according to studies. Then it levels off again at one percent a year.

In one-third of women, bad cells (osteoclasts) literally cut up the lacelike web of bone matter faster than the good cells (osteoblasts) can rebuild those webs. One doesn't feel a thing. The very stealthiness of this disease is its major threat.

Two factors determine a woman's risk of having significant bone loss during this transition. First, her genetic background, and here nature turns the tables on our Western beauty ideal. "I could look at a woman and bet her risks of osteoporosis—she's fair-skinned, very thin, a smoker, and has an early menopause—and usually she'll be symptomatic," says Dr. Lewis Kuller of the University of Pittsburgh School of Public Health.

The second factor is: How strong are the bones a woman has built at her peak? About one-third of American women of all ages are calcium-deficient. "The preoccupation of teenage girls is with thin thighs, not good bone, so they get into the habit of drinking diet soda instead of milk," laments Dr. Barrett-Connor. But generational differences here are striking. The frail women who are now immobilized in nursing homes are a different breed from baby boomers who are out there bouncing from work to gym in their nitrogen-cushioned aerobic shoes, popping calcium and snacking on veggies.

Porous bones, which lead to increased risk of fractures, are a major public health problem. One-third to one-half of all postmenopausal women—and nearly half of all people over age seventy-five—will be affected by this disease, maintains the National Osteoporosis Foundation. Forty percent of all women will have at least one spinal fracture by the time they reach eighty. And those who fall and fracture a hip have a 5 to 20 percent greater risk of dying within the first year.

Untreated, not only do older women die from the consequences of osteoporosis, but it often leaves older women frail, susceptible to falls and broken bones, as well as to the little tortures of hairline fractures in the bones they use for walking and bending—and this by their sixties. Later, in their seventies, osteoporosis makes it painful merely to sit on hipbones pulverized almost into powder; it keeps many women homebound, later even chairbound, and is one of the primary reasons an independent woman will finally succumb to nursing home admission.

"With osteoporosis, an ounce of prevention is worth ten thousand pounds of cure," emphasizes Dr. Zackson. "Frankly, we don't really have a cure."

What can a woman do to prevent this meltdown? A great deal.

If she starts in her thirties, she can do a tremendous amount with exercise and calcium supplements, increasing her bone density by 8 to 10 percent, according to Dr. Zackson. "It's like filling in potholes."

Later, during the period of accelerated loss, taking calcium supplements *alone* cannot undo the damage done by the loss of estrogen. And contrary to conventional wisdom, exercise *by itself* is also ineffective in preventing bone loss. These were the results of a study on prevention of postmenopausal osteoporosis reported in the *New England Journal of Medicine.* The best results were obtained when estrogen was *combined* with exercise: Bone mass was *increased* (and other symptoms—hot flashes and sleeplessness—improved) after three months.

What kind of exercise works for osteoporosis prevention? The dutiful pedaler on a stationary bike is not doing her bones much good, and swimming doesn't help, according to Dr. Richard Bockman, head of the endocrine department and codirector of the Osteoporosis Center at New York's Hospital for Special Surgery. The weight of the body has to be carried by the bones in order to stimulate bone strength. Brisk jogging requires a push-off that is much greater than one's body weight. The point is that one *needs stress* on that hip, and brisk walking can increase that stress in a natural way. "Everyone can walk briskly," encourages Dr. Bockman. "Or do serious walking on a treadmill at a tilt, which gives you both weight bearing and aerobic benefit." Exercise also increases flexibility and strength, so a woman is less likely to fall, and falls are the major cause of hip fractures.

A recent Georgia study shows that Tai Chi, an ancient Chinese meditation exercise with roots in martial arts, is extremely effective in the prevention of bone injury. People who practiced Tai Chi cut their falls by 47 percent, and in those who fall, the benefits of Tai Chi has shown to decrease fractures by 25 percent.

"Olympian estrogen users"—women who start HRT at menopause and remain on it to age eighty— show up in studies with the greatest protection of their bones and agility, and a 50 percent decrease in deaths as a result of hip fractures.

"But I'm already sixty—I missed the window," women often lament. "Isn't it too late for me to do anything to save my bones?"

The answer, happily, is no. Late use of estrogen has proven to be very effective in maintaining bone, as demonstrated by Dr. Robert Lindsay's study group at the Helen Hayes Bone Center. Women who start HRT at age sixty, after only ten years of use, can cut their continuing bone loss in half. Even if a woman starts using estrogen at age seventy, according to Dr. Bruce Ettinger, senior investigator at Kaiser Permanente's research division, as long as she stays on it for the next ten years, by age eighty she will enjoy almost the same protective effect as the Olympian user. Late use does not, however, build back bone already lost.

Today there are new standards by which bone density is measured. Most major American cities with a medical center or university have bone densitometer machines. Chemical markers have been discovered to help in identifying and treating osteoporosis. "Previously, a patient would get a bone density and then, a year or two later, would come back to see if they'd done well with the medicine they were given," says Dr. Joseph Lane, chief of metabolic bone disease at the Hospital for Special Surgery in New York. "Now we have chemical markers that allow us to get an answer within months as to whether these drugs are efficacious. There are markers that tell us if you are breaking down bone too quickly and markers to tell us if medication is working. The new tests are also predictive, indicating whether or not a woman can expect to make it to her sixty-fifth birthday without a fracture.

"We are also paying a lot of attention to body weight," says Dr. Lane. "We now know that people who have lost weight or have low weight are particularly at risk. We are starting to give caloric recommendations besides just calcium."

In August 1997 the Medicare Bone Mass Measurement Coverage bill was passed. The bill standardizes the way Medicare will be reimbursed for bone mass measurements. It will be implemented in July 1998.

Dangerous Breasts

A woman I'll call Sarah was brutally widowed in her prime of a dashing, beloved, prominent husband. She was left with a lovely apartment and a terrace garden which she let go to seed because she couldn't bear for several years to step out on it and be assaulted by painful memories. Sarah was a freelance commercial artist, and a very successful one. But in her misery she soon became blocked creatively and desperately lonely. Then to top it off—hot flashes. Hearing about "vaginal dryness" from her friends, she wondered if she would lose interest in sex before she was ready to enjoy it again. The terror of being identified as a menopausal woman overtook her. "And I'm single, so it matters."

Off to the plastic surgeon for a face-lift. Then to the gynecologist for something to "take away the embarrassment of these drippy hot flashes at dinner parties." She had to keep herself shelf-fresh if she was going to keep hope alive for recovering her creativity and her zest for finding a new partner in life.

Five years later she sat with me on her terrace and admitted her trepidation about taking hormones. "I have these dangerous breasts," she told me, stroking the unusually large, well-formed bosoms under her T-shirt, as if they had grown alien and were ready at any point to turn on her. "I have a history of breast cancer among the women in my family. But I also have osteoporosis in my family," she said miserably.

"I've been on hormones now for five years," she continued. "All I know is that once I started taking them, the flashes stopped and I had a feeling of well-being. And I looked okay. All that is important to me because I'm an older single woman. But am I doing something to my body that I'll kick myself for later?"

Like most of my educated and savvy friends, Sarah did not know that heart disease is the number one killer of women. A couple of years before, she'd had a bone density test and was told she was fine; the hormones were working.

Sarah has a new male partner now, and she has brought her terrace garden back to life. It's a place of delight where we sat that June day, surrounded by sprouting shrubs and her exquisitely cultivated roses, bathed in birdsong and a cool breeze. "It gives me such a lift when I wake up to come out here," Sarah said. She has become a happy, healthy, fully functioning, attractive, and sexual woman again. Hormones appear to be integral to her quality of life in her mid-fifties. What risk is she running by taking HRT?

A bombshell went off in 1997 when the most recent report on breast cancer came out of the twenty-two-year-old continuing Nurses' Health Study at the Brigham and Women's Hospital of Harvard Medical School. Those nurses who had been taking estrogen for ten or more years faced a 43 percent increase in the incidence of breast cancer.

"Ohmigod, those numbers are humungous!" was the reaction of most newspaper readers. This is a misleading figure, argues Dr. Michael Osborne, director of the Strang-Cornell Breast Center and chief of the Breast Service at New York Hospital. A more understandable number is this: If you had a two in a thousand chance of getting breast cancer at the age of fifty—without hormones—your chances would go up from two to three per thousand if you had taken estrogen for ten years. That is one extra case per thousand women—a definite, but small, increase in the risk of breast cancer after ten years of HRT.

Despite this increase, those nurses in the study who continued on hormones for more than ten years had a significantly *lower overall mortality rate.* "The basic conclusion is that for the hormone-using group as a whole, their overall risk of death was lowered," says Dr. Walter Willett, professor of epidemiology and nutrition at Harvard School of Public Health, one of the directors of the Nurses' Study.

A much more upbeat appraisal came in the same year, 1997, from an equally respectable academic study, which concluded that long-term hormone replacement therapy can boost life expectancy for most menopausal women. Researchers from New England Medical Center and Tufts University Medical School estimate that less than one percent of healthy perimenopausal women would fail to benefit from hormone therapy. Several other respected long-term studies of middle-class American women who have taken estrogen replacement for up to thirty years indicate they live longer—with a 20 to 40 percent reduction in mortality rate.

However, the duration of HRT use is critical, argues Dr. Willett. Taking HRT for two or three years, to get through the symptomatic period, poses no increased risk of breast cancer. "After five years of HRT, we begin to see some increase in breast cancer," says the Harvard researcher. "For women who stay on hormones for their postmenopausal lifetime, the risk of breast cancer becomes quite substantial."

Women are very well aware of the statistic that one in nine American women will be diagnosed with breast cancer. But this is a woman's risk *over a lifetime.* What is neglected, or generally unknown, is that the risk rises parallel with a woman's age. Two-thirds of all breast cancers happen to women beyond menopausal age. But the ones that shock us are the tragic one-third of cases that occur in younger women—mostly those in their forties.

Another startling statistic: alcohol consumption can increase a woman's risk of developing breast cancer up to 41 percent, according to a recent article in the *New York Times.* A new study that pooled data from studies of over 300,000 women in the United States, Canada, the Netherlands and Sweden, concluded that moderate to heavy drinkers (two to five drinks a day) put themselves at a risk comparable to having a family history of breast cancer or starting to menstruate before age twelve. The increase in risk for women who drank no more than one drink a day, however, was extremely small.

Women today are in the position to make more

nuanced decisions about their health as medical researchers learn more about the interplay of risk factors associated with breast cancer. So before you toss out your favorite vintage wine, it is important to evaluate your biological and psychological predispositions. If, for example, you have a family history of heart disease or you tend to be a hard-driving or intense person, but you aren't at high risk for breast cancer, it may be better for your health to enjoy a drink a day than abstaining from alcohol altogether. The protective effects of modest drinking on the heart have been well-established. On the other hand, a woman like Sarah who has a family history of breast cancer and has already been on estrogen for five years would be well-advised to drink only on special or social occasions.

In addition to age, the key risk factor is a family history of breast cancer. "When you're doing a family history, keep in mind that only a first-degree relative—mother or sister—poses an added risk," stresses Dr. Hiram Cody, a New York Hospital breast surgeon. "If it's a grandmother, aunt, or cousin, it's not nearly the same added risk, if any risk at all." Also, to be relevant, one's mother had to have been under the age of fifty when she developed the breast cancer. "It's a *pre*menopausal first-degree relative who contributes a significantly increased risk of breast cancer," affirms the leading researcher on menopause in Britain, Dr. Malcolm Whitehead. "Even with the worst possible family history," adds Dr. Cody, "a woman has no more than a fifty-fifty chance of getting breast cancer."

Researchers are now beginning to identify genes

that predispose a woman to breast cancer. BRCA-1 and BRCA-2 are the two main genes that have been discovered to date. Women who test positive for one of these mutations have up to an eighty percent chance of getting breast cancer. But not as many women as one might think are subjecting themselves to the cold scientific sentence that might be pronounced by genetic testing. Those properly concerned about confidentiality, the potential threat to their employability and insurance coverage, and especially the burden that carrying such knowledge would inflict upon themselves and their mates and children, may prefer not to know and take their chances.

What is usually obscured by our phobia about being stricken by breast cancer is the much more prevalent danger as we age:

Two out of three women will die of heart disease.

It is a well established fact by now that heart disease kills four times as many women as breast cancer does (see earlier chapter "The Cheating Heart"). The following is a startling scene between a contemporary woman recovering from breast cancer and her surgeon:

"Your CAT scan looks just fine, Ms. Brophy, where the breast tissue is concerned," the surgeon tells his fifty-year-old patient a year after her lumpectomy. "But from your bone density test, it looks like you're losing bone mineral pretty fast." He also knew that in Ms. Brophy's family history were blood relatives with heart disease. He suggested she consider going on a low dose of hormone replacement therapy.

"Are you kidding?" The patient sat up indignantly.

"I just put out the fires of breast cancer—why would I feed the flames now?"

The surgeon's next words amazed her.

"When breast cancer is diagnosed and treated early, as in your case, you can look forward to a nearly normal life span—you have a 90 percent survival rate. *The least of your worries now is dying of breast cancer.* Now you have the luxury of worrying about the much greater risks—heart disease or osteoporosis. One of them is going to get you first."

Dr. Michael Osborne is the surgeon quoted above. Given his lengthy experience as head of the Strang-Cornell Breast Center, he has learned to respect the need for estrogen replacement, even in some of his breast cancer patients who have family histories of heart disease, evidence of dangerous bone deterioration, or cholesterol levels out of whack. Dr. Osborne puts the question women must ask themselves in the simplest holistic terms:

"At the end of the day, are you more likely to be alive or dead if you take estrogen?"

He gives an answer with tongue in cheek. "You're more likely to be alive—and you'll probably be a whole lot happier."

What Is Your Lifetime Estrogen Budget?

༄

$\mathcal{A}$s a generation, boomer women carry an increased estrogen load, having been the first to use both oral contraceptives and estrogen therapy. It can be said that the more cycles a woman has, naturally and synthetically, the more estrogen she has in her system over a lifetime. The primates researcher Kim Wallen points out that for two thousand years most women cycled only two or three times before becoming pregnant, followed by several years of nursing, which again suppressed their periods; then they cycled again several times before their next pregnancies. Historically, then, a woman in her reproductive years may have had a total of forty or fifty ovarian cycles. The modern woman may have more than three hundred.

"So human females today are getting a very different pattern of hormonal stimulation," concludes Dr. Wallen. "Then, when they go through menopause, we are hitting them with another period of exposure to hormones that they never would have had in the past."

If you are still premenopausal, I would urge you to consider your lifetime "estrogen budget." Count the number of cycles you have had since you entered menarche. Then subtract the number of months you have supported pregnancies. Add debt to your budget to reflect the number of years you may have taken birth control pills, and further add the high doses of estrogen you may have added if you ever took fertility drugs. Overall, it appears that the risk of breast cancer from using hormones in menopause is highest for women who already tend to have excessive levels of estrogen. An overweight woman with lots of fat cells has a built-in risk factor. Other risk factors (in addition to the genetic predisposition) are early menarche, first pregnancy at a late age, or no children, all of which add to the lifetime levels of estrogen. Dietary risk factors include a habit of more than seven alcoholic drinks a week; possibly low levels of Vitamin A from a diet poor in green leafy vegetables and beta carotene; and a diet high in polyunsaturated fats. International health statistics point to a much higher incidence of breast cancer in countries where women eat a high-fat diet.

"We know that rural Japanese women who still eat a low-fat diet of vegetables, rice, and a little fish experience far less breast cancer than Japanese women who have become urbanized and now like steak and french fries," says Dr. Caldwell B. Esselstyn, Jr., a Cleveland surgeon who campaigns for health care "beyond surgery." He adds, "If the lobules and ducts of the breast are constantly being overstimulated by a high fat intake, which leads to higher production of estrogen, those tissues will be more likely to undergo cell changes leading to cancer." As former president of the American Association of Endocrine Surgeons, Dr. Esselstyn points to data showing that nations which consume greater amounts of fat per person have the highest mortality rates of breast cancer.

The fats that lessen the breast cancer risk are fish oils—like those on which the Eskimos exist—and canola oil or olive oil. The only safe margarine is one made from canola or olive oil. Look for the label: *No trans-fatty acids.*

Not only does a fatty diet add indirectly to the risk of breast cancer by increasing the estrogen level, but scientists have demonstrated in the laboratory that fat also has a direct effect on tumor growth *independent of estrogen.* Dr. David Rose at the American Health Foundation in Valhalla, New York, injected human female breast cancer cells into two groups of mice. He gave one group a diet of 23 percent corn oil, the same type of fat found in popular margarines. This high-fat diet both increased and accelerated the growth and spread of tumors as compared with the low-fat group. Rose's results, published in the *Journal of the National Cancer Institute* (October 1991) provide a compelling argument against high-fat diets to protect a woman from *both* heart disease and breast cancer.

"Nobody is arguing against estrogen supplements for the short term—the first three to five years of perimenopause and menopause," says Dr. Kuller, the public health expert at the University of Pittsburgh. "But for the long term, meaning ten to fifteen years, estrogen is drug therapy and should only be prescribed for women predisposed to osteoporosis or heart disease, or both."

But here's the rub. The key to hormonal protection against heart disease in older women, according to the Nurses' Health Study, was that the healthy women were taking estrogen *currently*. The risks and benefits of estrogen therapy on eight separate health conditions were totaled up in a thorough review by T. M. Mack at the University of Southern California. Stopping treatment with estrogen at the end of five years would produce a modest decrease in the risk of breast cancer. But it would also virtually eliminate all the benefits of long-term health enhancement—a Hobson's choice!

But at least we have choices.

Hormone Replacement Therapy:

Should I or Shouldn't I?

"Should I or shouldn't I?" is the question that dominates discussions about menopause among women, yet there is little agreement on the subject of hormone replacement therapy (HRT). Recent market research by drug companies suggests that women are still not well-educated about the long-term health consequences of menopause. The focus is still on hot flashes. A common attitude is, *The hot flashes go away anyway, so why would I need any kind of hormones?* There is little appreciation of the role played by estrogen in keeping a woman's bones strong, her heart healthy, and her memory sharp.

A few basic points need to be made at the outset.

⮑ Taking estrogen to replace what your body used to make is not for every woman. But it *is* for every woman to consider.

⮑ If you decide to use hormone therapy, you should

do so for a good reason, not just because your doctor hands you a prescription.

～ Many women say they are uneasy about taking drugs for something that is natural, not a disease. It is also not "natural" to live much beyond menopause. Most of our great-grandmothers did not live long enough to deal with the debilitating consequences of bone loss or heart disease. Exploring HRT as an option is a good way to start thinking about how to protect and enhance your health for the next thirty or forty years.

～ You don't have to make a decision for life. You make a decision that addresses the phase of menopause you're in right now. When you review it again next season, you may need custom-tailoring, just as you might let your skirts up or down.

～ If you do decide to try HRT, *expect* the first year to be trial-and-error. It is important to choose a doctor who recognizes the need to readjust the dose, or the regimen, or possibly changing the way it is delivered, (by mouth, through the skin, or vaginally), until your body responds optimally.

Women have a right to good, unbiased information about hormone replacement therapy. HRT is a health issue. Most women who take it do not do so just to stay youthful and sexy-looking. They take it because they are convinced it is good for their health and well-being.

Dr. Nita Nelson, a Los Angeles gynecologist, makes the case that estrogen is the only hormone that people are asked to live without. "If a woman is diabetic and doesn't have enough insulin, we don't say, 'Try to live without the insulin.' We know she's going to die sooner and that the years she has left will be poor unless we replace the insulin she is missing. The same goes for thyroid deficiencies."

So persuasive is the evidence of the many protective benefits of estrogen, a stunning 75 to 95 percent of American obstetrician-gynecologists say they would prescribe hormones to most of their recently menopausal patients. I asked one of the major researchers in Europe, Dr. Malcolm Whitehead, director of the menopause clinic at Kings College Hospital in London and president of the International Menopause Society, "If it were your wife, what would you tell her about coming to a decision?"

"I don't see it as much of a conundrum, perhaps because I'm a man," he opines. "If estrogens really do reduce coronary-artery disease death by fifty percent, that factor alone will swamp any other factor in the equation." Dr. Whitehead openly envies women for *having* a choice; men don't. "We are stuck from the time we're born to the time we die with arterial disease as a sword of Damocles hanging over us."

But women today are ready to take a more sophisticated approach to the "Should I or shouldn't I?" question. They just need to be walked through the latest data to make an intelligent, individualized decision.

Best Bets

$\mathcal{T}$he object for the HRT user is to get as much benefit as possible without adding measurably to her risks. This is achieved through moderation: by making a compromise between the maximum state of well-being at present—which usually requires high doses of estrogen and lower progesterone to make a woman feel just like she did before menopause—and the maximum protection of her body for the next three or four decades of life.

> *Women who receive the greatest benefit from HRT are those at high risk for heart disease and osteoporosis and low risk for breast cancer.*

Natural, plant-based estrogens have become the choice of many educated women. Foods rich in plant estrogens (soy products, lignans and isoflavones) could have similar benefits to hormones and may reduce the risk of breast cancer. These substances can be found in whole cereals, vegetables and fruits, soybeans, chickpeas, and other legumes. More promising designer drugs that address specific health concerns without adding to the risk of breast cancer are just beginning to be available (see chapter "New Frontiers in Treatment").

There are now at least a dozen different regimens recommended by doctors for combining the standard estrogen and progesterone. No two women respond the same way. One relatively new regimen has become popular: continuous, low-dose progesterone. The PEPI (Postmenopausal Estrogen/Progestin Intervention) trial found a woman doesn't need the "elephant gun" dose of progesterone routinely prescribed. Instead, a much smaller dose of a progesterone (2.5 mg), taken every day along with the estrogen, protected the uterus. Not only does this lower dose of progesterone minimize the uncomfortable side effects felt by many women, it frequently eliminates the return of periods, which is the main objection women have to remaining on hormones. This regimen usually smoothes out a woman's cycle so she doesn't have storms of hormonal highs and lows.

The American medical-pharmaceutical establishment persists in fostering suspicion of any "natural" compound that might alleviate symptoms—a shaky position given the many plants and barks from which major drugs like digitalis and even aspirin are derived. Fortunately, the women who designed the PEPI trial did not share this outmoded bias. In addition to testing the synthetic hormone products on the market, they pushed to include a natural compound meant to protect the uterus against cancer.

It is called natural micronized progesterone. Made from Mexican yams or soybeans, natural progesterone matches closely the chemical composition of the body's own progesterone. It is therefore less likely to confuse the body and lead to salt buildup, fluid retention, and hypoglycemia. *Micronized* means that the particles are finely ground and thus more completely absorbed. A continuous dose of the natural micronized progesterone in combination with estrogen every day turned out in the PEPI trial to be an excellent combination of hormones for women with a uterus: The regimen produced the best overall cardiovascular effect *and* proved to protect a woman against the risk of uterine cancer. What's more, the natural progesterone had fewer unpleasant side effects than the synthetic version.

This is the first time that a National Institutes of Health-funded scientific investigation into hormone therapy has ever given credibility to a natural compound. There is only one problem. American women can't easily get natural micronized progesterone, because it has not been approved by the FDA.

The Director of the Division of Reproductive and Urologic Drug Products at the FDA responded with tight-lipped evasiveness when asked why there has been such a delay in making this promising compound commercially available.

European women can easily obtain natural micronized progesterone from companies such as Schering-Plough, the German supplier of the PEPI trial. But a woman in the United States is out of luck unless she knows the names and numbers of the few pharmacies which sell it and can persuade her doctor to write a prescription.*

Why should women and doctors have to use an underground network to obtain a natural product when a government study, supported by their tax dollars, suggests it may be a safe, effective choice for combined hormone therapy?

---

*The Women's International Pharmacy (800-279-5708) or the Madison Pharmacy (800-558-7046), both in Madison, Wisconsin, are U.S. outlets for oral micronized progesterone (OMP), produced by Upjohn. It is also available through College Pharmacy in Colorado Springs, Colorado (800-888-9358) or Bajamar Women's Health Care in St. Louis, Missouri (800-255-8025). Wally Simons, the pharmacist at the Women's International, says that synthetic progesterone is from ten to a hundred times as potent as the natural micronized product. As the equivalent of 2.5 mg of Provera, he recommends from 100 to 200 mg a day of natural progesterone, preferably taken half in the morning and half in the evening.

Outgrown Worries

❦

Results from recent studies suggest a woman is in almost no danger of uterine cancer if she takes combination therapy: estrogen together with a natural progesterone or a synthetic progestin. But using estrogen alone *is* hazardous for a woman with a uterus. A surprisingly large number of the subjects given unopposed estrogen had to be taken off this regimen because of precancerous changes in the lining of the uterus. But University of Maryland epidemiologist Dr. Trudy Bush passed on relieving news for women who have been taking estrogen alone (often against doctor's advice). Two months after progesterone was introduced to their regimen, the lining of the uterus returned to normal.

Uterine cancer is a somewhat overrated concern, according to clinicians advising the Women's Health Initiative. Even women who do get endometrial cancer, and have appropriate treatment, live longer than women who *never* took estrogen and *never had uterine cancer*—a startling statistic. Nevertheless, using *combined* hormone therapy can diminish the concern of uterine cancer from the start.

Periodic ultrasound exams are a painless and reliable way for a woman to monitor both the health of her uterine lining and her ovaries. (Unlike mammograms, however, pelvic sonograms are usually not covered by most health insurance plans as preventive medicine.) If any thickening or unevenness of the lining is detected on ultrasound, then a more invasive evaluation of the endometirum can be done. Abnormal bleeding patterns may also be an early warning of precancerous changes in the lining of the uterus. However, this early sign does not always occur, warns Dr. Allen. Fortunately, the uterine lining is not difficult to monitor. A D&C can be easily performed and a woman can be taken off estrogen and treated with progesterone alone for awhile until her uterus settles down. There is a high cure rate with uterine cancer that is caught early.

The transdermal patch is an increasingly popular method of delivering estrogen to the body. A small adhesive bandage releases the hormone through the skin, with the advantage that it maintains a continuous, consistent level of estrogen in the system, like a time-release capsule. It is not metabolized through the liver and therefore has no impact on digestive diseases like ulcers. The FDA has approved transdermal patches as a treatment for menopause and osteoporosis. Estrogen delivered in this form, however, has not proven to be as beneficial in protecting against heart disease as estrogen taken orally.

At least one scientist with long experience in studying women who use hormone replacement therapy has unresolved questions about the transdermal patch. It can easily return a woman to a premenopausal state. That sounds desirable, and may explain why women are so enthusiastic about the patch, but there is another side to the story. According to studies done by Dr. Brian Henderson, the patch produces higher levels of the most potent form of estrogen (estradiol) than does Premarin, giving a woman almost as much hormone as she would have made herself. "The effect of that should be to make one's breast cancer risk go up substantially more on the patch than on Premarin," says Dr. Henderson. He points out that Premarin has been used for fifty years, while the patch has been widely available for only the last seven years.

Survivors of breast cancer are often doubly deprived. Until recently, it has been considered *verboten* to give hormone replacement therapy to a postmenopausal woman with breast cancer. Today, for a woman with a terribly symptomatic menopause, which may add to her depression over losing a breast, her quality of life must be weighed in the balance. Especially if she has had her ovaries removed, and has no circulating hormones at all, she may feel life is hardly worth living. Some physicians now offer such women the choice of taking a short course of HRT. (See chapter "Dangerous Breasts.")

There is considerable evidence by now that the drug tamoxifen may offer the benefits of hormone replacement therapy for the bones of a woman who has had breast cancer, while also reducing her risk of a recurrence. The problem with tamoxifen is it acts as an estrogen-like drug on the lining of the uterus, so the woman should have an annual ultrasound exam and vigilant monitoring of the uterine lining.

If you have had a precancerous condition in the cervix, not to worry; cervical cancer is not hormone dependent. Also, there is no evidence that estrogen replacement increases the risk of ovarian cancer.

Asking the
Right Questions

⌖

The debate over "natural" vs. "medicalized" menopause will only grow more vigorous as boomers come along. I was asked to give a talk in San Diego to women state legislators from all over the country on the subject of menopause. It was quite amazing: Four hundred busy political women stayed for several hours on the last Sunday of their conference to discuss every aspect of the Change. Many of them came to microphones to describe their experiences. One lawmaker from Minnesota told how a group of her peers in the state capital decided they weren't going to skulk around and hide their postmenopausal status—they were going to flaunt it. So they formed a bike club and rode to the statehouse wearing Day-Glo pink T-shirts with *THE HOT FLASHES* printed in black letters across the front. Finally, Betty Friedan took her turn and pooh-poohed the whole subject. Hormones were dangerous, and besides, who needs them? Drawing only on her own experience, she shrugged. "I *may* have had a hot flash, one hot flash, while I was giving a major speech in the middle of the Seventies."

But no one woman's genetic makeup should be held up as the model for abstinence from hormones, making the next woman feel lesser for having a different nervous system, a different metabolism, and different stores of hormones, just as she has different depths of pigment or strands of DNA in the tangle of her own creation.

Several studies indicate that women live longer if they are on estrogen. The Leisure World Study continues to follow 8,881 women, aged forty to one hundred one, all white and upper-middle class, in a Southern California retirement community. "The women who have used Premarin for the longest time have the lowest death rate," says Dr. Brian Henderson, who oversees the study. The more startling evidence from the 1991 follow-up is that *current users* who had taken estrogen for more than fifteen years, and were by then in their seventies and eighties, enjoyed *twice the benefit*—a 40 percent reduction—in their overall mortality.

"Women with symptoms certainly feel better when they take estrogen, and those in professional positions almost always feel they work and concentrate better," concludes Dr. Robert Lindsay. To make it easy for your doctor to take care of you during these years, know what you want. Here are questions to ask yourself so you can bring the answers to your doctor:

- Is there any evidence of osteoporosis in your family?

- Did your mother or a sister have breast cancer? How young was this first-degree relative when it was diagnosed? Was it estrogen-sensitive?

- Is there any family history of heart disease?

- Is there a family history of cancer of the uterus?

- Did you have serious PMS?

- How long have you been perimenopausal? (The longer it takes you to move from irregular cycles to no cycles, the more likely you are to have physical and emotional symptoms.)

- Rank order, on a scale from one to ten, what concerns you most about menopause—i.e., No. 1 might be the embarrassment of hot flashes in public, and No. 10 might be the fear of losing memory and concentration.

It's natural to want to put off asking ourselves such questions as long as possible, if not forever. But remember the goal that was stated at the outset of this book. You can now plan for your menopause the way you planned for your pregnancies.

Potential Benefits, Risks and Side Effects of Prescription Hormone Replacement Therapy for Menopause-Related Conditions

Potential Benefits	Potential Risks/Side Effects
ESTROGEN	
1. Prevents or reduces short-term effects of lowered estrogen, such as hot flashes and dry vagina.	1. Increases risk of uterine cancer if taken without a progesterone.
2. Reduces insomnia and improves deeper sleep, thereby helping to reduce irritability.	2. Appears to increase the risk of breast cancer if taken for many years.
3. Reduces risk of heart disease by as much as 50% (except for the vaginal dosage forms).	3. Increases water retention (bloating) and thus water weight gain in some women.
4. Prevents osteoporosis and, if the disease is already present, some estrogens can restore some bone loss.	4. Increases breast tenderness in some women.
5. Assists in maintaining a healthy genital area. Decreases risk of bladder infection. Protects against bladder incontinence and atrophy of the vagina.	5. Oral forms cause headaches and GI distress in some women.
6. May improve concentration and memory.	
7. May offer protection against Alzheimer's disease.	
8. Cosmetic effects: Keeps skin and hair looking younger longer.	

Potential Benefits	Potential Risks/Side Effects
PROGESTERONE	
1. Reduces any increased risk of uterine cancer caused from taking estrogen replacement therapy almost to the level of taking no hormones at all.	1. May reduce cardiovascular benefits gained with estrogen replacement therapy. Non-oral forms may have less of a negative effect than oral progesterone.
	2. Some regimens cause regular uterine bleeding similar to a menstrual period—more pronounced in women recently menopausal.
	3. May worsen mood (PMS-like symptoms), although progesterone and non-oral forms may have less of a negative effect than oral progesterone.
TESTOSTERONE	
1. Increases sex drive in selected women, particularly following surgical removal of ovaries.	1. Overdosage may not improve sex drive and can cause agitation and/or depression, acne, as well as masculinization (facial hair growth, muscle weight gain, etc).
2. Increases energy in some women.	2. May reduce estrogen's heart health benefits.
	3. Safety over the long term has not been established.

Regimens of Prescription Hormone Replacement Therapy Commonly Used in the U.S.

U.S. Trade Name	Generic Name	Route of Administration
ESTROGENS		
Premarin	Conjugated equine estrogens	Oral, vaginal cream
Estrace	Micronized 17-beta-estradiol	Oral, vaginal cream
Estraderm, Vivelle, Climara, Alora	17-beta-estradiol	Skin patch
Estring	17-beta-estradiol	Vaginal ring
Estratab	Esterified estrogens	Oral
Ogen, Ortho-EST	Estrone estropipate	Oral
PROGESTERONES		
Provera, Cycrin	Medroxypro-gesterone acetate	Oral
Micronor, Norlu-tate, Aygestin	Norethindrone acetate	Oral
Prometrium (coming in 1998)	Micronized progesterone	Oral
*Crinone	Micronized progesterone	Vaginal gel
Progestasert	Micronized progesterone	Intrauterine device
*Not FDA-approved		
COMBINATIONS		
Prempro	Conjugated equine estrogens and medroxyprogesterone acetate	Oral (in single pill)
Premphase	Same as Prempro	Oral (in two separate pills)
Estratest	Esterified estrogens and testosterone (an androgen)	Oral (in single pill)

Charts are useful for general reference, but no two women's risk-benefit profile is the same. Both the Nurses' Health Study and the New England Medical Center/Tufts University Medical School study point out that the balance of risk and benefit really depends on who is taking hormones and for how long.

Most to Gain from HRT

A woman at high risk for heart disease and osteoporosis and low risk for breast cancer.

Least to Gain from HRT

A woman who has no family history of heart disease or osteoporosis; who has always had calcium in her diet and hasn't been a long-term smoker or heavy alcohol user or had an eating disorder; who exercises, is not overweight, and during perimenopause a baseline bone density shows her bones are sturdy. This woman does not have a lot to protect. "We did not find any substantial reduction in overall mortality among women whose risk of heart disease is already low," reports Dr. Walter Willett, one of the investigators in the Nurses' Study, "because the protective benefits of estrogen on heart disease were offset by the increased risk of breast cancer."

Highest Risk in Taking HRT

- Immediate relative has had premenopausal breast cancer

- Extensive use of birth control pills or fertility drugs

- No children

- Overweight

- Drinks more than seven drinks per week

- Breast biopsies have shown "proliferative changes." (Ask for your pathology if told you have benign breast disease.)

The Weight-Gain Conundrum

❧

*A*mong those women who are given prescriptions for HRT, half of them either don't take the hormones as prescribed or throw out their pills within less than a year.

Why?

According to my medical colleagues on the advisory board to the Women's Health Initiative, the two main reasons women resist or discontinue taking hormones are fear of breast cancer and weight gain.

Women invariably blame hormones for whatever weight gain occurs once they start taking HRT. The number one side effect named in a survey by *Prevention* magazine was weight gain, reported by 60 percent of women who took hormones.* What most of us don't understand (or don't want to accept) is that a dramatic change in metabolism takes place in both

---

*Cathy Perlmutter, Toby Hanlon and Maureen Sangiorgio, "Triumph Over Menopause," *Prevention,* August 1994.

women and men in middle life. In women that change corresponds coincidentally with the menopause transition, which usually gets blamed for it.

"Women preserve their fat-free mass quite well, relatively speaking, up to about age forty-eight or forty-nine, with little age effect," according to Eric Poehlman, Ph.D., associate professor of gerontology at Veterans Administration Medical Center in Baltimore, who has studied hormonal changes related to food, diet, and exercise in many different populations. "But there's a significant change after age forty-nine, about a 4 or 5 percent decline in fat-free body mass. And that is in healthy women *not* on HRT."

The PEPI study confirmed this conclusion. The women who gained the most weight during the three-year trial were those who took no hormone therapy at all. And over large studies it has been found that women who take estrogen tend to weigh less and to be thinner than women who do not. We also know that women who take HRT are more likely to be college-educated and have above average incomes. Indeed, studies have shown a striking correlation between high social and economic status and a woman's weight.

The higher a woman's socioeconomic bracket, the lower on average is her weight.

(Incidentally, the opposite is true for men. Among men, the higher their socioeconomic bracket, the higher their weight tends to be.)

Dr. Louis Arone is director of the Comprehensive Weight Control Program at the New York Hospital-Cornell Medical Center. "The short answer is, we don't know why some women gain weight when menopause begins, but it's very common. Abdominal fat is the usual complaint. We think it's because of the change in hormone status. You can't spot reduce it or make the fat go away by doing sit-ups."

One of his patients, a community fund-raiser, went through menopause relatively late. She started hormones and blew up from 115 pounds to 135 pounds in just a couple of months. She came to Dr. Arone and asked, "Could this be the hormones? What do I do?"

"We temporarily stopped the hormones, put her on a balanced low-calorie, low-fat diet—lots of vegetables, moderate protein and carbohydrates, and less than 30 percent fat. We talked to her gynecologist, and she lost about a pound a week. It took four or five months, but she got back to 115. Now she's back on HRT. It's the progesterone that promotes the weight gain," Dr. Arone reported. Hormones can also cause bloating—from salt and water retention—and they can cause weight gain.

It's much easier to prevent obesity than to correct it. Not everybody can get back to their premenopausal silhouette, so expectations should not be too high. The real point is, it's much easier to curb the weight gain that might be brought on by menopause if a woman anticipates the Change.

The good news is that a woman can wipe out the age effect on her weight—with exercise and resistance training (with weights). If she starts regular exercise—especially if she started before she enters menopause—she can prevent muscle mass from turning into fat.

"I would strongly recommend that women going into menopause exercise regularly—both aerobically and with weights," says Dr. Arone. "If you can do it three days a week, that's the minimum. Anything more than that is terrific."

Diet modification is a necessity as we get older and burn calories more slowly. Another recent report from the Nurses' Study warns that it is not so much the quantity of fat in our diets that determines a woman's risk of suffering a heart attack. The villains are saturated fats, found in meats, whole milk and cheeses, and a new villain known as "trans-fats," found in most margarines, including corn oil margarine, commercial baked goods and deep-fried foods— like french fries—prepared with hardened vegetable oils like Crisco or lard.

So what kind of fat and cooking oils *can* a person use? Pure vegetable oils, like corn or safflower, that is in liquid form—the label will read "polyunsaturated" or "monounsatured". (When food manufacturers hydrogenate these vegetable oils, to make them last longer, they become trans-fatty acids and promote heart disease.) Even better are canola oil or olive oil. Extra virgin olive oil carries other mysterious nutrients for the heart that give it a long track record as a healthful staple in the Mediterranean diet.

Do I Have to Stay on Hormones Forever?

ॐ

One of the scare statements often repeated is that hormones will only put off the inevitable. "A woman who starts on hormones will have to stay on forever because if she stops, all the menopausal symptoms will return with a vengeance," a prominent New York gynecologist told a new patient. This "express train" scenario is false, says Dr. Lila A. Wallis, a New York internist with forty years of clinical experience and many older patients who have grown into their sixties under her care as users of hormone replacement therapy.

"In the very early menopause, women require larger doses of estrogens in order to control their symptoms," says Dr. Wallis. "As they get older, the estrogens can be cut down and the patient is more tolerant of the decreased dose."

The one action to avoid is to go off hormones "cold turkey." The operative generalization is this: *The more abrupt the drop in estrogen, the more severe are the symptoms.* This explains the severity of symptoms often reported after a hysterectomy or during a sudden, stress-related menopause, just as it explains the flare-up of symptoms that may occur if a woman who's been suppressing them for a decade with HRT abruptly discontinues the hormone bath to which the body is accustomed. There is a simple way to avoid this problem: tapering off. Dr. Wallis advises her older patients to note whether or not hot flashes or any other symptoms resurface when their regimen of replacement hormones is, at first, slightly reduced. As symptoms subside, the regimen may be further reduced or discontinued. The body has a chance to adjust over time.

A New Regimen for Postmenopause

$\mathcal{W}$hat about the idea of stepping down the dose gradually as a woman passes the ten-year mark as an HRT user?

Dr. Bruce Ettinger of Kaiser Permanente in Oakland, is a respected researcher who supports the growing trend of lowering the dose of HRT to the minimally effective level. Women and their doctors have been given the impression that only .625 mg of estrogen is effective. However, results from a recent double-blind, placebo-controlled two-year study, indicate that half-strength estrogen (0.3 mg) can still increase bone mass (though not as much at .625 mg) and provide some protection against heart disease, while greatly reducing the accumulated risk of breast cancer.

It has taken decades for scientists and clinicians to understand how estrogen really works in the body. (Earlier, the scientific community feared that estrogen replacement would endanger women's hearts!) And now, just as the full estrogen story is being told, a whole new chapter in the treatment of menopause is beginning to be written—at first, in glowing terms.

New Frontiers
in Treatment

❧

$\mathcal{A}$ whole new class of drugs and alternative therapies are entering the menopause marketplace with the jawbreaker name of SERMS—selective estrogen receptor modulators. "Designer estrogens," as they are nicknamed, are said to work like estrogen to protect the bones and heart while canceling out the added risk of breast or endometrial cancer. Sound too good to be true?

Designer estrogens do open up a whole new approach to protecting the health of postmenopausal women. They fill in the gap for women who want to protect their bones and who cannot risk standard estrogen replacement. But their impact on the heart and the brain are still uncertain.

Raloxifene, manufactured by Eli Lilly, is the first SERM to be rushed to market, under the trade name Evista. Given fast-track approval by the FDA, it was released in late 1997 only for the prevention of osteoporosis. The company plans to promote the drug heavily to address the emotional issue of women's fear of breast cancer.

Clinical trials showed that Evista builds bone, although to a lesser extent than either estrogen or Fosamax, the current drugs used in treatment of osteoporosis. But it is too early to say Evista will reduce the incidence of breast cancer, as initially reported. SERMS do not stimulate breast tissue or the lining of the uterus, as estrogen can. However, the safety information on Evista was gathered in clinical trials on 10,000 women taking the drug for up to thirty months—hardly long enough to evaluate how much or how long it would affect a woman's natural risk of getting breast cancer as she ages. Studies of the effects of Evista on cholesterol levels were conducted for only six months, and showed that the drug significantly reduced LDL, or "bad" cholesterol, but did not increase HDL, or the "good" cholesterol. And it has no effect on the lining of the blood vessels, as does estrogen.

SERMS do not help with memory or concentration. Moreover, this early version is known to increase the number of hot flashes, which are usually triggered by the brain's attempt to deal with falling hormones. That raises another question: Just as it acts as an anti-estrogen on the breast, might Evista act as anti-estrogen on the brain?

"With SERMS we have nothing yet in terms of information or material to show that there is long-term protection against heart disease," says Dr. Wulf Utian, professor of reproductive biology at Case Western University and founder of the North American Menopause Society. "And though we have a whole new family of SERMS developing, raloxifene being the first one, even then it is not showing any effects that we can see on cognition or enhancement of any brain function."

This is only the beginning of possibilities in the evolution of a very promising new category of drugs that may offer women in menopause the protections they need without the current risks. Stay tuned into SERMS.

The third most common reason women stop using HRT (after fear of breast cancer and weight gain) is an acute sensitivity to progesterone. "Usually women who are progsterone-sensitive have a history of depression, even low-level, or some anxiety disorder," says Dr. Jeanne L. Leventhal, clinical assistant professor of psychiatry at Stanford Medical School. "Taking progesterone makes women with untreated low-grade depression or anxiety disorder feel worse during menopause—and they don't know why."

One future possibility for women who are hypersensitive to progesterone and unable to take other forms of the hormone is a gel called Crinone. It is a natural progesterone developed by Columbia Laboratories and licensed by Wyeth Ayerst. Crinone comes in a similar form to Replens, the vaginal moisturizer, and sends progesterone to the uterus to protect from endometrial cancer. Very little of this form of progesterone is absorbed into the bloodstream and therefore does not affect moods in a negative way.

Approved by the FDA in July 1997, Crinone is prescribed in a 4 percent dosage, containing 45 mg of progesterone, for the treatment of secondary amenorrhea, the absence of a monthly menstrual cycle. Some physicians have found it beneficial as a hormone replacement for progesterone-sensitive menopausal women. But this use of the drug for this purpose has not been approved by the FDA, and Wyeth Ayerst awaits further studies by Columbia.

Natural estrogens can also be obtained through diet. Foods rich in plant estrogens, known as phyto-estrogens, could have some of the benefits of hormone replacement therapy and almost none of the side effects. These substances can be found especially in soy products, and to a lesser degree in whole cereals, vegetables and fruits, chickpeas and other legumes.

Making Your Choice

If we approach this journey with optimism, determined to become informed consumers of health information and choosy about the physician who will work with us as a partner, we can live and love and work and cope quite well. Here are three important ways to think about the passage through menopause:

First, consider the time you have left to live—one-half your *adult* life. If you have the good fortune to reach menopause, you have a responsibility to educate yourself on how to preserve your physical and mental well-being so that your older years can be vigorous and independent. Think of going for the long haul. Take a life review of where you have been, the parts of yourself you have already lived out, and those yearnings you left behind as a girl. How can you put play back into your life? How can you turn your talents and life skills to caregiving in the broader, even worldly sphere? What adventure of mind or heart or bold personal challenge would your ideal future self dare to take? Consult her; then follow her lead!

Second, find the information you need to help you manage your menopausal transition. A woman's wellness center may be sufficient to answer your questions. Most doctors will tell you if you ask them honestly: How many women do you treat over the age of forty-five? (That will tell you how interested or experienced the physician is in treating menopause.) Ask the doctor to describe menopause to you. Then ask questions. If your inquiries are brushed off with pat or curt answers, walk away.

There is a simple blood test a woman can ask for that is quite reliable in determining whether or not, and at what stage, she is in menopause. One should ask to have one's LH and FSH measured, along with the level of estrogen. (FSH, a follicle-stimulating hormone, and LH, a lutenizing hormone, are responsible for ovulation and under the control of estrogen and progesterone.) If the FSH and LH are both high, in the presence of low estrogen, it is indicative of menopause.

If you have risk factors for osteoporosis, it is important to have an osteoporosis screening. (See pp. 181–182 for details.)

Be an inquiring, even challenging partner, not a passive follower of doctor-as-God. Decisions on how to plan for the health and well-being of your next thirty years or more cannot be made in a twenty-minute visit with your doctor, any more than you would decide on the purchase of an expensive car in that time. Expect a year of trial and error.

Third, take charge of the transformation. This is the maximum opportunity for transformation in a woman's life. She no longer has to be a pilot fish swimming in someone else's wake or a mother hen distracted by caregiving demands. This is the time to stretch and strut and shout about whatever engages her mind and spirit. For a woman who has worked all her life, this transition may demand that she stop pushing herself so hard professionally or inviting so much stress. The postmenopausal years invite streamlining, shucking the nonessential in favor of full focus on the passion of one's life. More time devoted to deepening one's spiritual practices is a natural preparation for coming to terms with future health crises. A wisewoman will make time to contemplate things eternal and to appreciate the life she has.

Cultural
Catch-Up

❧

Doctors Coming out of the Dark Ages

∾

So often women say, "I'm waiting for my doctor to tell me what to do."

Lamentably, few doctors are well informed about menopause. Medical schools spend no more than half a day on the subject, if that, I am told by doctors. Many assume the vaguely described symptoms are psychological in nature. Since physicians are temperamentally disposed to helping people, they, too, feel frustrated at the state of scientific ignorance about women's health in the middle years.

"You don't need to know about that yet" is one standard answer women are given. The doctor pats her on the head, and out the door she goes with her migrainous headaches, ill-defined blues, or unexplained fatigue. More commonly, she won't even bring up menopause, and her gynecologist won't either. Some women spend the next three to five years making the rounds of internists, neurologists, even psychiatrists, with no resolution, because they all ignore the obvious.

The experience of a busy professional political activist in Washington is emblematic. Noticing her periods were scanty and intermittent, and feeling uncharacteristically draggy, she went to her internist and plunked down three hundred dollars for a complete physical. She was forty-nine. The physician took a considerable amount of blood for tests. The results shed no light on her condition. Only when the activist talked to a woman friend who asked, "What about your estrogen level?" did the lightbulb flash on. She realized her doctor had not taken any hormone levels. He had never even mentioned menopause.

"The most important change going on in the body of a forty-nine-year-old woman was never addressed," she says, chagrined at her own passivity. "Doctors treat our bodies as though we're the same machines as men, and we're not."

A woman's own signs are her best guide as to whether or not she is nearing menopause or what phase of the long transition she might be in, and whether it is causing her problems. But in order to recognize those signs, and deal with each appropriately, *we must be educated.* It will not do to retreat behind the defense, *If I don't acknowledge it, it doesn't exist.*

Educated women have begun to let their doctors know they want a *dialogue* about menopause—a safe environment to ask questions, and explore options— not to have hormones thrown at them. Physicians and medical centers have responded. Doctors (125,000 of whom are women today) are fighting over which specialty is best able to treat this newly identified and lucrative patient group. But one doctor can't know everything about all of the short- and long-term health issues involved in the biological and psychological transition of menopause. Women who have problems should be encouraged to seek help from different professionals if they need it, says Dr. Fredi Kronenberg, the director of menopause research at Columbia-Presbyterian Medical Center.

In 1991, while serving as Surgeon General, Dr. Bernadine Healy marshalled the government's backing for the Women's Health Initiative (WHI). The largest clinical study of women's health in American history is investigating whether women who use artificial hormone therapy for many years are actually better-protected or at greater risk from such post-menopausal health hazards such as heart disease, breast cancer, colon and rectal cancer, and fractures from osteoporosis. The earliest results will not be reported before the year 2000. Until then women and their physicians will have to make a compact to act as partners.

Some obstetrician-gynecologists find the menopausal woman an unappealing patient. She isn't going to have any more babies. Apart from a hysterectomy, there is little chance she will require surgery—the moneymaking part of the practice—but she can be expected to complain about vague symptoms and ask questions for which even the sympathetic physician has only unsatisfactory answers. With candor, a dedicated female gynecologist describes the attitudes of many of her male colleagues: "They find us tedious because we're going to take up their time, and threatening because we're smart and we're grownups—we don't want any of their bullshit."

This is not to imply that all male gynecologists are dismissive or that all female gynecologists are sympathetic. Women who have felt the necessity to deny their femaleness in order to "pass" in male-dominated medical schools and hospital settings may disassociate from menopause entirely, and they can be quite brutal with women patients who bring them a grab bag of complaints.

The busy doctor of either sex is likely to take an incomplete family history of the factors that impinge on menopause. Just how cursory these conversations can be is illustrated by the experience of a well-known columnist and her sister, both hard on age fifty. They consulted the same gynecologist in the Boston area to ask what to do. Despite their genetic likeness, one was told she was a good candidate for hormones. Her sister was cautioned not to take hormones. It turns out that the sisters had emphasized different subjective fears.

Dr. Mathilde Krim, the indefatigable AIDS activist and former pioneer in interferon research, relates another typical story. "Very early on in my life I was shocked by the great indifference of male doctors to the health problems particular to women," she says, recalling the unnecessary secondary suffering of a woman cancer patient at Memorial Sloan-Kettering Cancer Center. Dr. Krim had been called into the group of male physicians discussing the woman's case: Her cancer was of the lung. The patient was asked what other medications she took. "Estrogen," she volunteered.

"That's the first thing to cut out," the men ordered. "Why, if it makes her feel better?" demanded Dr. Krim. "It was absurd. The poor woman had all these problems with her lung cancer, and now she had to suffer hot flashes on top of it." But the male physicians were gratuitously adamant. And of course, the patient did not dare to raise a complaint.

Today, let's hope she would put up a fight.

The
Hysterectomy Trap

꙳

*E*ach year about 560,000 women in the U.S. undergo hysterectomies. In fact, the hysterectomy is the second most common surgery for women in America, more than double the rate in most European countries.

A mere 11 percent of these menopause surgeries performed in the U.S. are done in response to a cancerous growth. Notwithstanding, some gynecologists urge women to consider a "prophylactic hysterectomy." That is, to undergo major surgery *on the chance* that at some future time she might develop cancer in her reproductive organs.

A Seattle divorcée brags about solving the whole dilemma by having just such an elective hysterectomy at the age of forty-one. "My doctor was a yanker instead of a saver," she quips. "But I wasn't going to use the equipment anymore, I didn't want it. I'm glad I got rid of my ovaries."

It may sound like a nice midlife housecleaning, but

that brings us to another myth about the Change: If you have a hysterectomy, you bypass menopause.

A case in point is the story of a Rochester woman I interviewed, a college professor in the social sciences. Virginia, who requested anonymity, was regarded by her family and friends and colleagues as a "super-coper." At the age of forty-seven, she separated from her husband. She went into perimenopause at the same time, but she didn't know it.

Then came the all-too-common admission: "I thought, because I'd had a hysterectomy, I wouldn't *have* a menopause." Virginia never asked her doctor. And her doctor, a woman GP, said nothing to enlighten her.

"I was agitated all the time," she recalls. "I thought I was losing my memory. I had night sweats and blurred vision. Sometimes I'd be so fatigued my legs would fold underneath me climbing up the stairs." Two or three times a week after work, Virginia would drive an hour and a half to Buffalo. There, unrecognized, she could sit in a shopping mall and cry.

Only recently, in Virginia's fifty-second year, did her doctor measure her hormone levels. She announced: "Virginia, you're finished with menopause."

It was the first time the subject had come up.

If both a woman's ovaries are removed, she will go into instant menopause. Twice as many women who have a hysterectomy today, compared to twenty years ago, also have their ovaries removed. For a woman with a persistent ovarian tumor, it is common and necessary to have at least one ovary removed. However, before having both ovaries removed, a woman should be warned that the abrupt and total, rather than gradual, shutting down of ovarian function can be devastating, placing her at risk of serious depression.

It also extinguishes sexual desire. Unless a woman immediately starts hormone replacement therapy and commits to remaining on the medication indefinitely, she will have all the symptoms of menopause, whatever her age. What's more, early surgical removal of the ovaries *doubles* the risk of osteoporosis. If you lose your ovaries at age thirty, by the time you reach age fifty, your *bone age* may be seventy. Yet doctors often neglect to warn a woman that the surgery can have such lifelong effects even after the body heals.

I ran into this same high-handed attitude in a heavily utilized menopause clinic in the heart of London. "In a postmenopausal woman, the ovaries are of no use anyway," a doctor replied dismissively.

I expressed alarm. Wasn't this extreme? The doctor was ignoring a very important continuing usefulness of the ovaries. Although a woman's ovaries stop producing estrogen, in postmenopause, they continue to produce a significant amount of testosterone. And testosterone strongly influences a woman's sexual desire and energy.

"The concept that the ovary burns out is not true," claims one of the experts on the postmenopausal ovary, Dr. Howard Judd at UCLA. A study that did take the trouble to consider the impact on sex life following a hysterectomy found that between 33 and 46 percent of the women whose ovaries had also been removed complained of reduced sexual responsiveness.

"This uterus looks a little bit tired," a male gynecologist told a forty-year-old North Carolina woman.

"Guess we'll take her out." It was typical of the attitude among some doctors that the uterus is little more than a nuisance. Since this patient was a housekeeper, without all the fancy scientific words to defend the tired "her," all she could do was "fight to keep my uterus."

Fibroids often lead women to unnecessary hysterectomies. These benign growths are found in 20 percent of all women. Here is a typical scenario from the Massachusetts Women's Health Study of twenty-five thousand women, aged forty-five to fifty-five, from all socioeconomic levels:

A woman who is perimenopausal but doesn't know it goes to her doctor to report heavy bleeding. "Is this the Change?" she asks. He tells her she's too young for the Change, but she'd better have a D&C. The study investigators follow up eighteen months later. By now, the woman has gone in for two or three D&C's, which haven't stopped the bleeding because it wasn't abnormal—it was normal perimenopause. But by now the woman is so scared, she ends up having an unnecessary hysterectomy, which only serves to bring on menopause sooner and with far more severe symptoms.

Now, what could this woman have done instead? A simple office biopsy of the lining of the uterus could document any evidence of premalignant changes. Or, she could have a hysteroscopy, an examination that allows the physician to look inside the cavity of the uterus and see if there is a polyp. If there is still doubt, she could take a three-month course of hormone replacement, to see if the dysfunctional bleeding is resolved.

Some women with fibroid tumors do have clear

indicators for hysterectomy: first, rapid growth of the tumor which may be a sign of cancer developing in the fibroid; second, uncontrollable bleeding; third, fibroid size so large that other organs may be compromised; or, finally, intractable pain.

At some level we *know* when the Change begins to come upon us. The sense of unease or disequilibrium is something that women feel, although it remains incomprehensible to those who have not experienced it. Isn't it amazing that women should allow organized medicine, filtered through a male perspective, to tell us how we feel? (How many men know what it's like to be one week late? Or two weeks early while you're teaching a class in a white suit?)

Medical breakthroughs in this century have given us the gift of greatly extended life spans; now attention should be turned to ensuring *healthier* life spans. And that means women must become informed, active consumers of good health care. But because up to the present day we have accepted a way of thinking that denies or denigrates this epic change in our bodies and the exciting new vistas it can open in our minds, we have failed to demand that decent scientific research be done.

Our tax dollars have supported massive research on heart disease among men (while leaving women out of those clinical trials entirely), but our national health institutes can give us little definitive data about the long-term impact of the body's postreproductive state on women's health. The National Institutes of Health has spared only 13 percent of its revenues to study women's health. Medical schools still use terms such as *the weeping of the uterus* to describe menstruation, assigning emotions to a bodily organ because it wasn't fertilized by male sperm that month. The classical medical terminology for menopause is *ovarian failure*.

Another way of seeing it would be as *ovarian fulfillment*. One has put in thirty or forty years of ripening eggs and enduring the hormonal mischief of monthly cycles, on the chance that a child is wanted. Enough, say most women in middle age. We're ready to move on now, to find our place in the world, free of the responsibilities of our procreative years. It's time to take risks and pursue passions and allow ourselves adventures perhaps set aside way back at twelve or thirteen, when we accepted the cultural script for our gender that ordinarily downplayed those dreams. It's time to kick up some dust!

The
"What About Me?"
Syndrome

ess privileged women assume that menopause is just another burden of being a woman and simply bear it, though not grinning. But the class differences are glaring. The population tapped for the rare studies has been almost exclusively white, well educated, and motivated to take care of their health preventively. The vast majority of women in lower socioeconomic groups have no idea of the long-term health issues related to "the Change." They are so accustomed to bleeding and having cramps and premenstrual tension that when they hit menopause they just shrug and say, "Here we go again—male doctors treating me like I don't matter a damn."

That was Kate McNally's first reaction. A fifty-five-year-old secretarial assistant in a medium-size Long Island town and mother of four, Kate went to her gynecologist complaining of heavy bleeding. After a questionable Pap smear, a cone biopsy was done, followed by a D&C. She was put on estrogen and told to have a mammogram. The results weren't conveyed to her for two months: A lump had been found. Of course, at first she blamed the hormones. But the great majority of breast tumors, including hers, are slow-growing. Her disease had probably been developing, undetected, for several years. The irony is, many women do not bother with a mammogram *until* they consult a doctor about indications of menopause. If a tumor is found, the culprit may look like hormones, but is probably the result of more careful medical surveillance.

After two lumpectomies, Kate was taken off estrogen forever. She was bedeviled by menopausal symptoms no one could tell her how to relieve. "I feel betrayed," she said softly. "I've always put others before myself. By this age I have more money to work with and more leisure time with the kids gone. I should have the energy to do the things I've always wanted."

I asked what things she had looked forward to.

"Getting a decent night's sleep."

This modest expectation was betrayed by the dull film over her blue eyes. "You go for years with little babies waking you up all night. Then the teen years when you can't sleep for worrying because they're out in your car. And now *I'm* the one awake all night!" She laughed hard. Her husband seemed wonderfully supportive, and Kate was determined to cope with this stage as she had with other trials in the past.

A treatment alternative for women like Kate might be tamoxifen, an estrogenlike drug that is protective of the heart and prevents bone loss at the same time as it protects the breasts against cancer. There are a number of tamoxifen trials underway around the country. Tamoxifen is not a perfect alternative since it does increase the risk of uterine cancer, but that risk can be easily monitored and corrected.

Kate's sister, Bindy, was only forty-two and very attractive, with long, curly red hair and a sugar-doughnut figure wrapped in shorts and a T-shirt. But already she was wrestling with the emotional preamble to menopause. "I used to be the no-worry type. Just leave the house, go to the beach—nothing ever bothered me," she said. "I lost my temper but once in a blue moon." Suddenly she was a virtual powder keg. When her son didn't come to the table until his dinner was cold, she jumped up in such a childish rage she knocked over a chair. "Everybody looked at me as if I had three heads."

Veteran gynecologists affirm that some women can have physical symptoms from even slight changes in the amount of estrogen produced. Sensors in the brain that control emotions pick up a signal when there is an erratic production of either estrogen or progesterone. In a person whose nervous system is finely tuned, these sensors overreact, triggering brain-chemistry changes and emotional symptoms.

Every morning, as a waitress in a busy coffee shop, Bindy has to stroke hundreds of people who haven't had coffee yet. "The doctor told me to stop smoking, cut down on cholesterol, and avoid stress. Hah, avoid stress! How?"

She knows she is being grouchy and impossible. "But I can't control it. And I'm afraid if I take this estrogen, then *I'll* have lumps like my sister."

* * *

Women like Kate and Bindy are often caught in the middle between caring for aging, fragile parents and dealing with the lingering financial dependence of children. Many experience the "What about me?" syndrome. They are not accustomed to nurturing themselves. But even as they are encouraged by books like this to pamper themselves through this transition, Western society is making more demands on them today than ever. Most middle-aged Americans today still have living parents, a change in family dynamics with no precedent in history.

Since most women are going to have to take care of an aging parent or parent-in-law, more and more women will be put on "the daughter track," possibly for a decade or more, just as they are emerging from the "mommy track." Traditionally, it has been middle-aged women who are depended upon to do the work of unpaid caregiving for the disabled elderly at home. But women now also fill nearly half the paid positions *outside* the home. At just the stage when they expect to enter the most focused and productive period of their working lives, with their children grown and gone, they may not be able to carry the new double burden of elder-caregiving and full-time career. Many will have to switch to part-time jobs, forfeit promotions, or quit their jobs altogether, unless they demand reforms in public policy and decent eldercare. The cruel choice for a growing number of menopausal-aged women will be: Do I take care of my mother in her old age, or provide for independence in my own old age?

Across Color, Class, and Culture Lines

⚜

Cross-cultural studies of women and menopause reveal that the change of life is experienced differently depending on one's cultural assumptions about aging, femininity, and the societal role of the older woman.

Anthropologist Mary Catherine Bateson points out: "In many societies women are granted a greater degree of freedom after menopause than they were permitted in their reproductive years. This may be because women no longer represent a risk of 'pollution,' or no longer need to be sequestered as sex objects through whom their husbands might be dishonored." Indian women of the Rajput caste do not complain of depression or psychological symptoms of menopause since they are freed from veiled invisibility and at last are able to sit and joke with the men, reports anthropologist Marcha Flint. Furthermore, in some traditional societies such as Iran's, women only come into their own when they have an adult son. Bateson describes how grown-up sons literally pay court to their mothers, visiting them with news and flowers.

Women in Asian countries report fewer and less severe symptoms than menopausal women in the West—even though the mean age at menopause is the same across the board (slightly over fifty-one years). These findings were presented at the Sixth International Congress on the Menopause, held in Bangkok in late 1990. The study included women from Hong Kong, Malaysia, the Philippines, South Korea, Taiwan, Indonesia, and Singapore.

In China, where age is venerated, menopausal symptoms are rarely reported. Similarly, anthropologist Margaret Lock observed after studying a thousand Japanese women that 65 percent of them consider menopause uneventful. The Japanese language does not even have a word for hot flashes. (A report in *The Lancet,* however, describes "sinking spells" among Japanese women, rather like the swooning of Victorian women.) However, the virtual nonexistence of hot flashes in Japanese women is *not cultural,* according to Lock. It is due primarily to their different diet and the vigorous physical exercise built into the life of even elderly Japanese women. Their bloodstreams show high levels of soy (a source of estrogen) and calcium from a fish-dominated diet. And because most Japanese women have small kitchens, they walk or bike daily to the shops and hand-carry groceries back home, routinely enjoying a much higher degree of exercise than most middle-class women undertake in the West. As a result, menopausal women in Japan are not as prone to menopausal health problems as Western women are; they have a much lower incidence of heart disease, osteoporosis, and breast cancer. Although only two percent of Japanese women take hormones, they are the longest-living women in the world.

In America, youth and desirability go hand in hand, and the role for the older woman is uncertain at best. Ours is also an overweight, underexercised culture, particularly in the upper age brackets. Very few roles or jobs in this information age demand that American women over forty exert much more physical effort than opening their car doors and microwaves. But although menopause in the U.S. is defined primarily in hormonal terms, cultural attitudes do cut deeply.

Although I did not undertake a "scientific" sampling of American women's menopausal experiences, I did interview more than one hundred women from diverse racial, class, and educational backgrounds. I discovered that the women who enjoy a boost in postmenopausal status and self-esteem are those who perform roles in which intellect, judgment, creativity, or spiritual strength is primarily valued—politicians, educators, lawmakers, doctors, nurse-supervisors, therapists, writers, artists, clergywomen, etc.—while women whose worth was earlier judged primarily on their looks and sex appeal—movie actresses, performers, many full-time wives and mothers—are diminished in status. Women who build close bonds to grandchildren may make themselves indispensable, and often enjoy a tender and playful intimacy that brings them closer than they were to their own children.

African-American women in general are more likely than white women to pass through menopause with no psychological problems. Why? I wondered. After this book was first published, a friend and former professor of adult development, Clementine Pugh, gathered together a fascinating discussion group with twenty accomplished African-American women, most of them educators with advanced degrees. They agreed that African-American women do not measure their femininity and sensuality only by how they look. Nor is their self-worth attached to their age—how young they look. A great deal of a black woman's sexuality is defined by her spiritual strength, a strength dictated by her cultural history.

Middle-class black women come out of matrilineal tradition, and they gain in prestige and self-esteem as they enter middle age. They definitely *do not* give up on themselves as sexually desirable or desirous. What's more, sensuality, for the African-American woman, is not associated with the European-American anorexic body type. Stop and think about the many great older black women entertainers who sing and shake and bring the house down—from Moms Mabley and Ma Rainey to Della Reese, Patti Labelle, and even the opera superstar Jessye Norman. The older and broader they are, it seems, the more shamelessly lusty they can be. In short, menopause is more readily accepted as an integral part of life.

Women of color, however, do have their own physical vulnerability—fibroid tumors—far more common among African-American women than in white women, according to the National Black Women's Health Project. This higher incidence remains unknown, since African-American women are generally excluded from clinical studies, or are unidentified by race. Since fibroids often lead women to unnecessary hysterectomies, Frances Dorey, chair of the project, says "Black women are lucky if they even make it to menopause with a uterus."

Pamela Pilate, a nurse with the giant California HMO, Kaiser Permanente, conducts menopause education classes in downtown Los Angeles. When I asked her if she had noticed any cultural differences among her students, Pilate said something startling even to herself:

"The white women attend my menopause class. The black and Hispanic women come to my hysterectomy class." Women of color or low income who present an assigned Medicaid doctor with symptoms common to the "fearsome forties"—heavy, clotted bleeding and cramps—are most likely to be steered toward a hysterectomy. By the time they are referred to a nurse-counselor like Pamela Pilate, they already have a date for surgery.

As an African-American woman herself, Pilate is dismayed by how passively many of her patients surrender their reproductive organs. "When women of color have female problems, their usual reaction is to wait," the nurse-practitioner reports. "It's denial or fear." Lack of basic medical knowledge about their own bodies also plays a large part. As Pilate notes, "White women look for other alternatives—nutrition, herbs, or less invasive surgical procedures for removing the benign growths." By the time the black women come to her hysterectomy class, they have waited a long time to see a doctor, and they are either in pain or suffering from heavy bleeding or urinary problems. The fibroid may have grown to the size of a grapefruit. When Pilate inquires if their surgeon also plans to remove their ovaries, most of the women have no idea. "Usually, they don't know the function of their ovaries."

Pilate's lecture stresses that hysterectomy is a last resort. She also emphasizes that as a woman approaches menopause, uterine fibroids usually shrink if she doesn't take HRT. "But the women I see have a cut-and-dried attitude. 'This is part of life, what else? Let's get it over with.'"

Postmenopause and Coalescence

$\mathcal{O}$nce the menopausal transition is complete, a woman enters a new state of equilibrium. Her energy, moods, and overall sense of physical and mental well-being should be restored, but with a difference. Think of it as discarding the shell of the reproductive self—who came into being in adolescence—and coming out the other side to *coalescence*.

It is a time when all the wisdom a woman has gathered from fifty years of experience in living comes together. Once she is no longer confined to the culture's definition of woman as a primarily sexual object and breeder, a full unity of her feminine and masculine sides is possible. As she moves beyond gender definition, she gains new license to speak her mind and initiate action.

Whereas people in their late thirties and early forties are commonly pursued by a frantic hurry-up feeling—as if everything they have missed out on must be seized immediately or lost forever—the fifties open up the youth of Second Adulthood. What may have been seen as a dead end is now perceptible as a gateway to years ahead that spread out like a brand-new playing field.

"I spent a large part of my early adult life on logistics—just getting from point A to point B with three young children and no money," said an animated fifty-nine-year-old schoolteacher, describing her postmenopausal change of outlook. "Now, with no responsibilities and three functioning children who are off on their own, it's a liberation that is difficult to explain. It's emotional, physical, financial—total."

We have a second chance in postmenopause to focus on the thing we most love and to redirect our creativity in the most individual of ways. We must make an alliance with our changing bodies and negotiate with our vanity. No, we are never again going to be that girl of our idealized inner eye. The task now is to find a new future self in whom we can invest our trust and enthusiasm.

Today's "coalescents" are mapping out a whole new stage of life. Despite all the idiosyncrasies of this age group, common refrains emerged in the stories given by American women in their fifties:

"Making choices is so much easier" was a comment echoed from coast to coast.

"You don't get your period, *and* you don't have to panic when you don't," summed up a West Coast woman.

"You don't have to play the girl game anymore,"

said an attractive divorcée who has let her hair go gray. "But it's still all right to be vulnerable and allow yourself moments of weakness. Now it's *your* choice."

The "empty nest" that psychoanalytic theorists warned would leave us feeling useless and irrelevant turns out not to register as a main concern in large-scale contemporary studies. When women mentioned it at all in interviews with me, it was usually with relief or relish.

"After being liberated from keeping those five long-legged sons filled up, a new world opened up to me as I approached fifty," said a southern woman who had happily fulfilled the duties of a full-time wife. "One of the kids said, 'Mom, what are you going to do with yourself now that we're all gone?' I said, 'Hon, I don't know, but count on it—I'm going to have fun!'"

"The freedom of middle age is fantastic!" exulted a former homemaker who loves her new life as a real estate maven. "Now *Mom* can lie down before dinner. Or I can pay somebody else to do dinner. Or I don't have to have dinner at all."

"My marriage has found new dimensions," says Lisa Corletto, a fifty-year-old woman. "I actually take pleasure in preparing myself with scents and oils like a twenty-year-old. My husband constantly tells me how different everything is and how wonderful it is to come home. My creativity has soared, my outlook is youthful, and my future? Well, nothing is impossible!"

A great discovery of the fifties is the *courage to go against*—against conformist behavior and conventional wisdom. A woman can at last integrate the rebellious child of former days. Social psychologist Bernice Neugarten reports that as women move into later life, they become more accepting of their own aggressive and egocentric impulses and are unencumbered by feelings of guilt.

Given the added status and confidence of the postmenopausal state, women are in an optimal position to voice their convictions and make a powerful public impact. An initial sense of timidity may give way to relief and excitement as the new older women realize there are still many "firsts" ahead. Once they stop clinging to a life and conditions that have been outgrown, they can stake out their freedom at last.

"I'm not pulling my punches like I used to—I'm saying more of the things I really think," boasted a beautiful Rochester woman, now sixty-eight, who has remade herself into an organizational management executive.

"I grew up mechanical, I could fix a flat or repair the roof, but I always deferred," admitted a well-built African-American woman of sixty who takes care of a three-family house. "Now I don't need anybody to tell me how."

"You have the whole spectrum of intellectual capacity to draw upon," enthused a physician who left conventional medicine and is enlivened in her late fifties by practicing nutritional medicine.

Such comments hint at the welcome change of perspective as women come through the disequilibrium of menopause into the stage of mastery that follows it—a passage that is not cause for remorse but for celebration. In fact, in my previous studies of life stages on sixty thousand adult Americans, women in their fifties reported a greater sense of well-being than at any previous stage in their lives. A considerable body of psychological study data has accumulated since then confirming that women are *least* likely to be clinically depressed in middle age.

Extra-Sexual Passions

✑

$\mathcal{A}$t a small conference organized by Group Four on "The New Older Woman," held at the Esalen Institute, prominent American women from diverse backgrounds and professions were invited to share viewpoints on what it's like to be energetic, ambitious, optimistic, and over fifty in today's America. Most said they had negotiated the passage through menopause with a minimum of difficulty. The happy little secret they shared was that they had enjoyed the best sex of their lives during and just after menopause, between the ages of forty-five and fifty-five. Granted, their generation had been sexually repressed in youth, but these were also women of a generation totally unschooled in what to expect of menopause. The usual comment was that they were "too busy" with career, personal relationships, or family to dwell on the physical or psychological accompaniments to the Change.

Participants now in their sixties or older agreed

that there came a point, sometime in their fifties, when they had to let go—or at least stop trying to hang on to—their youthful image and move on. Although painful at the time, they discovered a reservoir of renewed energy and exhilaration—a "kicker."

As each one described her personal struggle, a common denominator emerged and the group hit upon something profound: The source of continuing vitality was to find your passion and pursue it, with whole heart and single mind. It is essential to *claim the pause* and find this new source of aliveness and meaning that will make the years ahead even more precious than those past.

For several of the women the passion was to correct an ignored community or societal wrong. Harriet Woods, for example, the former lieutenant governor of Missouri, had lost a Senate race and turned to creating a brand-new political institution, a think tank at the University of Missouri. She went on to become president of the National Women's Political Caucus, the only bipartisan national membership organization that recruits, trains, and supports women for elective and appointive office. "Age no longer has the same relevance it used to have," she affirms. In both roles she was able to pursue her passion: helping women learn to use their power and transform society.

Others had found more private passions: going back to school to finish a degree, writing a book, or the pursuit of knowledge in a special field for the pure pleasure of it.

The older woman with fewer resources often feels isolated, even cheated. Just as she feels free to pursue personal goals, her husband may be going into decline or physical dependency; returning children may try to manipulate her into remaining chief cook and laundrywoman; divorced or ailing parents may cramp her financially. But although these realities might sound like arguments against risk-taking at this time of life, in fact they make it all the more essential to dare new explorations.

Vi Beaudry defied all these assumptions about the "trapped" menopausal woman, and it wasn't because she had plenty of money or fancy degrees.

"It was my *husband* who had himself a menopause, okay?" she explains. "Some pause. He sat down in front of the TV and didn't get up for the next ten years. And it wasn't paid retirement."

On her fifty-seventh birthday, Vi had a revelation: She did not need a man to live, and she wasn't living with a man. Vi went back and gave her husband an ultimatum. "I would like for you to contribute something to the running of the household by September first." When the date came and he demurred, Vi filed for divorce.

Now sixty, Vi runs the community arts festival, sits on several community boards, and is one of the most lusty, healthy, outspoken people in town.

How one *welcomes* postmenopause and consciously prepares for the new freedom it offers, makes all the difference in reaping the benefits of the stages beyond. Anthropologist Mary Catherine Bateson counsels: "Say to yourself, I'm going to start a new life. It could be a stage of expansiveness or withdrawal. It could be a time of introversion or of worldly adventure."

In preparing for a smooth postmenopausal passage, it is useful to look to the most vital women of later age and how they have met the challenges of later-life passages. Cecelia Hurwich, one of the participants in the Esalen conference, conducted a study on women in their seventies, eighties, and nineties for her doctorate at the Center for Psychological Studies in Albany, California. The women selected had remained active and creative through unusually productive Second Adulthoods and well into old age. What were their secrets?

"They live very much in the present but they always have plans for the future," Dr. Hurwich said. They had mastered the art of "letting go" of their egos gracefully so they could concentrate their attention on a few fine-tuned priorities. They continued to live in their own homes but involved themselves in community or worldly projects that they found of consuming interest. Close contact with nature was important to them, as was maintaining a multigenerational network of friends. And as they grew older they found themselves concerned more with feeding the soul than the ego.

Surprisingly, these zestful women were not in unusually good physical shape. They had their fair share of the diseases of age—arthritis, loss of hearing, impaired vision—but believing they still had living to do, they concentrated on their abilities rather than on what they had lost. Over the ten-year course of the study, most were widowed. This hardship, like so many others they had endured, they turned into a source of growth rather than defeat. Frequently they mentioned in conversation, "After my husband's death I learned to . . ."

Every one of them acknowledged the need for some form of intimacy. They found love through sharing the most natural of pleasures: music, gardening, hiking, traveling. Several spoke enthusiastically of having active and satisfying sex lives. One woman, when asked how she felt about the automatic assumption that women in their seventies and eighties lost all interest in sex, answered after a long pause:

"This is how it is for me. I've become a vegetarian, but every once in a while I want a piece of red meat. And I go out and get it and eat it and enjoy it."

Wisewoman Power

❦

*W*omen who no longer belong to somebody now can belong to everybody—the community, a chosen circle of friends, a worship group, or even to the world—by virtue of contributing knowledge or creative insight or healing gifts. The elder women who survived in ancient or tribal cultures became sources of experience and wisdom and were often venerated as shamans with healing powers. As the influence of female deities increased steadily up to about 500 B.C., the role of medicine man was assumed by medicine woman. "The fact that women were shamans during this period indicates they had entered into the most authoritative and honored ranks of healers," writes Jeanne Achterberg in *Woman as Healer.*

The key to finding a new sense of empowerment in the Second Adulthood comes from moving through the crisis of aging to *generativity.* This entails a profound shift from pouring all one's energies into procreation, raising one's immediate children, or into one's own advancement, toward feeling a voluntary obligation to care for others in a larger sense.

Margaret Mead regarded postmenopausal zest as a widespread phenomenon. In the book *Composing a Life,* Mary Catherine Bateson describes the shattering series of blows her mother experienced before she reached a complete "renaissance." Her adored husband had left the marriage, her closest colleague died, and she spent several years improvising a life as a divorced professional mother of a small child.

But between the ages of forty-five and fifty-five, as Bateson pieces together the famous anthropologist's history, "She seemed to become prettier, she bought a couple of designer dresses from Fabiani for the first time, and I think she started a new romantic relationship." Boldly Dr. Mead returned to the field at the age of fifty-one: She boned up on languages and went back to New Guinea, forging a major intellectual new start with groundbreaking research on social change published in the book *New Lives for Old.*

In fact, hormonal changes may partly explain why so many women describe a vastly increased store of energy after menopause, while some men move toward despair and decline. A good deal of the energy of a younger woman goes into producing enough of the hormone progesterone to sustain a possible pregnancy. Postmenopausal women no longer suffer from the handicap of continually fluctuating levels of progesterone. Menopause also puts an end to the mood swings of the menstrual years.

"Do you know how you feel a week after your period ends—like you could climb mountains and slay dragons? That's how a postmenopausal woman feels all the time, if she's conscious of it," says Elizabeth Stevenson, a Jungian analyst in Cambridge.

Stevenson had a year of hot flashes, which she relieved with acupuncture, and by the age of fifty-two broke through to a state of postmenopausal zest. "It's both physical and psychological," she says. She doesn't have the same energy level she had at twenty-five, but she monitors and shepherds her energy so that her working days begin at eight and end at eight. If she eats right and exercises, she says, the consciousness of the wisewoman is always with her.

Emptying
and Refilling

❧

$\mathscr{M}$astering the physical and psychological challenges of the Change might be seen as a necessary exercise, forcing us to look ahead and accept the new perspective coming into view. Each major life passage entails emptying and refilling. It is particularly literal, and poignant, during menopause. There is first the gushing, like the reddening of a tree as it blazes in autumn with a flaming canopy before going dormant. As we move into postmenopause, we are emptied of the menses that has dominated our reproductive phase. We are reduced to basics, forced to lie fallow. Within that emptiness, watered by tears over the surrender of our magical powers of birthing, we can discover our greater fertility.

The greatest boon of menopause is that it forces us to tune in to our body's needs and quirks. It is, after all, the house in which we will dwell for the rest of our days, and we will be comfortable in it only if we learn how to turn down the stress on our heart and keep the mineral turning over in our bone. A new balance must be struck between output and input.

What is needed for replenishment?

For some women it's the decision to take off on a four-day weekend every six weeks—to climb a mountain, look at the sea, or simply drop out with music or books—whatever it takes to empty one's cares and find a centering calm. For others, the Change is the signal to give up unhealthy eating habits, stop smoking, invest in serious exercise, and learn what their body needs to feel good. For those who are already exercise habitués, they may need to balance aerobic exercise, which is demanding of the body, with yoga or meditation.

I wasn't ready to be fifty until I was fifty-two. By then, I had made several logical steps up to a new perspective. If we allow the mind to expand and explore higher realities, the body follows. At some point over the course of those two years I suddenly knew, with utter certainty, that as I grew older I was going to get better. I invited my body to accept that new reality. I could begin to visualize, positively, the vast unmarked territory from here to my eighties. The journey excited me. I felt almost giddy, like a pioneer. And by then, I had sorted out the practical aids and rituals that belonged in my long-term survival kit.

My personal choice, predicated on a family history of severe osteoporosis and no cancer, was to start hormone replacement therapy. It took me, however, a couple of years of experimentation before I found the right preparations and regimen to complement the peculiarities of my body chemistry. I am very glad I had the patience to stick it out. But as I approach ten years of hormone use, I am experimenting with reduced-strength estrogen. At first, foolishly, I stopped HRT cold turkey. After the first couple of weeks it was "Hello!" to hot flashes again, then to tossing around at four A.M. with night sweats. Drinking a glass of warm soy milk before bed helped, as did the collection of herbs in Dr. Corsello's Meno-Pak. But clearly, it is wiser to reduce one's usual dose of estrogen very gradually. And soon it may be attractive to supplement half-strength estrogen with one of the SERMS for osteoporosis protection.

At the same time I am disciplined about daily exercise to keep my muscles tight, my bones strong, and my mental acuity and memory pumped up with oxygen and those wonderful endorphins. Every woman is different, but for me, the daily ritual that keeps the motor purring is to down a dollop of Royal Jelly on awakening, to use nothing but natural oils on my face, and to bounce off (with the beat of rock oldies in my Walkman) to take a jog on nice days or work out with free weights and a treadmill. If time is short, I jump up and down on a tiny portable trampoline. I try to balance these weight-bearing efforts that are so good for the bones with meditation or a yoga class; it puts some elasticity back into sore sinews and stops the beat of urban life long enough to allow one to center.

Like many women who found motherhood deeply satisfying, I now find myself drawn irresistibly to gardening. Whether it's planting pots of petunias on a balcony or digging a fragrant herb garden, perhaps pitching earth and nurturing tender blooms is our subjective way of replacing the joy of growing babies. I plant a new tree each year and take pleasure in watching its progress like a child moving through school. And whenever I'm in London, I look for offbeat bulbs for my Shakespeare garden; they never fail to amaze and delight me when they finally sprout.

Vitamins are vital at this age—C, E, B-6, and of course calcium enriched with Vitamin D. Since natural sources of calcium are best, I take low fat milk on my cereal and in my coffee, and often a glass of warm soy milk at night to put me to sleep. Biannual vaginal sonograms and annual mammograms and biannual bone density checks are part of my discipline. Happily, I have *built* bone since I turned fifty with this regimen of exercise and hormone replacement. Finally, for husbanding my energy (and energizing my husband) I find that getting away together every six weeks or so for a long weekend adds immeasurably to the sweetness of life. And with our children grown, we can take off at the drop of a hat!

It has been a long road, but having "rounded the horn," I feel rekindled, high-spirited, and at home again inside my body. According to my husband, I look better, even younger, than I did when the journey began (thank goodness for the nearsightedness of middle age!). I am not the same me anymore. I am an older woman, that is true. The energy is not the same jumpy fits and starts I had as a younger woman; it is deeper, sustained, and with naps for refreshment, it seldom fails me. The outlines of my future self are coming into focus—and I like her. She is diligent but not so driven. She dares me to follow my purest instincts in what I think and read and write, rather than what is expected or externally valued. Do serious work and try to make a difference in the world, yes. But she won't let me neglect that part of myself that wants to play and rediscover the harmless things I did as a young girl— like getting lost in the woods. She dares me to take off on adventures. I've decided I'll go along on the trip with her, believing that the best stages are yet to be.

The magic charm, finally, is very simple. It is to say to yourself, *No, I won't go back. And I won't try to stay in the same place, inside the same skin. I will go forward. I have the courage to take the next step.*

I believe it is vital to develop a future self in the mind's eye. She is our better nature, with bits and pieces of the most vital mature women we have known or read about and wish to emulate. If we are going to go gray, or white, we can pick out the most elegant white-haired woman we know and incorporate that element into our own inner picture. The more clearly we visualize our ideal future self, admire her indomitable skeleton and the grooves of experience that make up the map of her face, the more comfortable we will be with moving into her container.

An inspiring public model of wisewoman power is Elizabeth Cady Stanton. As one who pursued justice for women well into her eighties, Stanton was living proof of her belief, which was eloquently recounted in her autobiography:

The heyday of a woman's life is the shady side of fifty, when the vital forces heretofore expended in other ways are garnered in the brain, when their thoughts and sentiments flow out in broader channels, when philanthropy takes the place of family selfishness, and when from the depths of poverty and suffering the wail of humanity grows as pathetic to their ears as once was the cry of their own children.

Postscript

To mark my own rite of passage through menopause I gave myself a few days alone in the mountains. I wanted to honor my graduation into the new stage of Second Adulthood and to reward my body for all the days it had already served me. On the last day I awoke after a full refreshment of sleep on a nearly empty stomach and opened the curtains to a dazzling sight.

The moon hung full over the hills. Unhurried by the day's first light, she reveled in her fullness. I went outside to sit in contemplation of her, and we faced each other in utter equanimity: She who had pulled the tides of my inner sea for 450-some months, powerfully, capriciously, violently, now had relaxed her hold on me and left my waters calm as a lagoon after a tropical storm. Emptied, I sat there in the twig-brushing breeze and savored the quiet aliveness that had come to me at last.

The moon began to sink. I felt pulled to hike once more up a mountain considered sacred by shamans

277

who once ministered to the Indians of this valley. Even then this mountain radiated a spiritual energy that drew those most subtlely attuned. Here the shamans marked rites of passage and performed rituals for birth and rites of fertility. It seemed an apt place to create my own ritual.

On the approach to the mountain my senses were quickened by each patch of herbs—the snap of sage, the tickle of thyme, the melancholy of rosemary, and what was that? The swoon of honeysuckle? Soon the scents were left behind as the bare rock and silver stubble of the foothills asserted their elemental simplicity. No frills here, only endurance. The wild herbs and grasses and desert flowers have the look of all healthily aging things: silvery gray, with strong roots, their flexible stems able to bend in the storm, their flowers calculated to bloom in the fissures between. All that is most creative and startling in life springs up in the cracks between.

As I followed the spiraling path up the mountain, lifting out of myself, I felt my inner world merging with the outer world. It was a world of silences, broken only by the munch of footfall on the crumbled earth and the sucking of Santa Ana winds. The moon was still in place. All at once the sun carved a dipper out of the opposite mountain and ladled its liquid gold down the face. The pure energy was almost overpowering. A sparkler of red and green spun for a few seconds in a mirrored circle beneath the great ball.

Then I sat for an undeciphered period of time in meditation on the brow of the far mountain. Honor the mellowed silence in you, *I thought.* Mark these moments when you are aware of not doing, not wanting, not preparing for the next activity, but simply filling with the moment. *The more still I became, the more I was able to feel the earth traveling beneath me. I could see the sun hung over one horizon, ravishing, while behind me, the moon was fading. The cymbals of day and night hung in perfect equipoise. The wind quieted.*

Then all at once I felt a surge of energy. Warm, whirling, giddy, it moved upward. A sense of such exultation filled me. It was as if the hourglass had been turned over and the crystals of creative energy were flowing in reverse—from womb to mind. I couldn't wait to get back to my laptop, my writing . . . my passion.

We are all pilgrims together, finding our way, but the markers we lay along the trail will beckon future generations to even longer lives. Let us mark the way well. Filled with new life and license, let us bring the cymbals of light and shadow together and begin again.

Index

Abelin-Sas, Graciella, 112
Achterberg, Jeanne, 267
acupuncture, 163
adrenal glands, 54, 123, 153
adult life cycle, xvii, 7-8, 10
African-American women,
    250-53, 260
aggressiveness, 62
aging
    of baby boom generation,
        xi, xvi-xvii, xix, 37, 41
    and brain function, 145-
        46, 147
    and breast cancer, 186
    cultural differences in,
        248-49, 251
    and estrogen loss, 16, 42-
        43
    and estrogen therapy, 36
    and health, 9-10
    vs menopause, 9, 18, 43,
        51
    and sexual desire, 21-22,
        112, 117-21
    stigma of, xvii, 7, 32, 36-
        37, 101, 130
    and weight gain, 216-18
agnus cactus herb, 162-63
Albright, Madeleine, 62
alcohol consumption, 166,
    186-87, 191, 214
Allen, Patricia, xxiv, xxv, 22-
    23, 24, 26, 29, 34, 37,
    70, 74, 87, 92, 135
allergies, 165
All in the Family, 11
Alzheimer's disease, 141,
    143

American Psychological
   Association, 85, 102
androstenedione, 57
animal studies, 56-57
antioxidants, 147, 163
anxiety, 86, 106, 129, 137
Arone, Louis J., xxvi, 217-18
arteries, narrowing of, 91
Ayurveda, 164

baby boomers, xi, xvi-xvii,
   xix, 28, 37, 41, 67, 87,
   107
Bachmann, Gloria, 127
Bajamar Women's Health
   Care 203n
Ballinger, C.B., 95, 98
Baltimore Longitudinal
   Study of Aging, 143n
Barrett-Connor, Elizabeth L.,
   154-55, 168, 178
Bateson, Mary Catherine,
   17, 248, 264, 268
Beaudry, Vi, 264
Bellifemine, Susan Sangillo,
   73
birth control pills, 93, 190,
   191, 215
black cohosh, 88
bladder problems, 91-92
bleeding. *See* menstruation
bloating, 25, 82, 218
blood acidity, 163, 166
blood pressure, 174, 176
blood test, 105, 155, 229,
   234
blood vessels, 91, 176
Bockman, Richard, 90, 180
Boggs, Pamela P., xxv
bone density test, 24, 113,
   154, 181-82, 184, 188,
   273

bone fractures, 173, 179
bone loss. *See* osteoporosis
brain
   and aging, 145-46
   and estrogen loss, xix, 43,
      85, 135-44
   hypothalamic regulator in,
      164-65
   and menopausal
      symptoms, 52, 135-37,
      246
   natural boosters for, 147-
      49
   and REM sleep, 98
   stimulating, 146
BRCA-1/BRCA-2, 188
Break of Day (Colette), 53
breast cancer, 34, 106, 157,
   168-69, 173
   and alcohol consumption,
      186-87
   and estrogen, 175, 184-85,
      186, 188-93, 206
   family history of, 187-88,
      210
   and fat intake, 191-92
   treatment of menopausal
      symptoms after, 206,
      245-46
breasts
   benign disease, 215
   cystic, 85, 92, 160
   tenderness in, 25
   tissue atrophy of, 92
breathing, deep, 88
Brown, Tina, xiv
Buhai, Suzanne Rosenblatt,
   41
Bush, Barbara, 83
Bush, George, 54-55
Bush, Trudy, xxv, 14-15, 42,
   204

Cai, Denning, xxvi, 162
calcium, 163, 178, 179, 214, 249
Callil, Carmen, 120-21
cancer, 9, 236-37
 cervical, 207
 endometrial, 23, 204, 226
 ovarian, 207
 uterine, 34, 173, 204-05, 246
 see also breast cancer
careers. *See* workplace, menopausal women in
cervical cancer, 207
Chase, Sylvia, 68
chemotherapy, 83, 106, 110
childbirth
 and life expectancy, 109
 and postpartum depression, 108
 postponement of, 15, 108-09
Chinese medicine, 88, 160, 162, 166, 167
cholesterol level, 91, 173-74, 176, 225
Chopra, Deepak, 164, 165
Ciba-Geigy, 129
cigarette smoking, 22, 166, 173, 175, 178, 214
Close, Glenn, 30
coalescence, 13, 257-74
Cobb, Janine O'Leary, 119, 142
Cody, Hiram, 92, 187
Colette, 53
College Pharmacy, 203n
Composing a Life (Bateson), 268
concentration, xix, 20-21, 25, 43, 97, 130, 138, 139, 141

cone biopsy, 244
control, loss of, 155-58
Corletto, Lisa Menzies, 17-19, 259
Corsello, Serafina, 159-62, 166, 272
cramps, 25, 252
Crinone, 226-27
cultural differences, 248-53
Cytoxan, 106

D&C, 205, 241, 244
depression, 23
 clinical, 97
 and estrogen, 97-98, 108, 137
 and hysterectomy, 102-03
 as malaise, 95-97, 98
 in mothers' generation, 47, 94-95
 postpartum, 108
 and sleeplessness, 98-99
 and stage of life, 6
 temporary, 47, 95, 103
DHEA, 83
Diamond, Marion, 146
diet, 10, 71, 147
 and breast cancer risk, 191-92
 estrogen sources in, 163, 200-01, 227, 249
 fat in, 163, 175, 191-92, 219
 for heart disease prevention, 173, 175
 for menopause symptoms, 89, 163, 166, 249
 weight loss, 113, 154, 182, 218
Ditkoff, Edward, 97
Ditropan, 92

doctors, 16, 18, 22
  ignorance about
    menopause, 233-34,
    242-43
  selecting, 229
  specialists, 234-35
  see also gynecologists
dong quai, 88, 162
Donner, Rebecca, 46-47
Dorey, Frances, 251-52
dream research, 98
Dwyer, Cathy, xvii

eggs
  donor, 110
  and ovulation, 14, 84
Ehrenreich, Barbara, 63
Eli Lilly company, 224-25
Ellerington, Mike, xxvi
emotional problems. *See*
    depression; mood
    swings
empty nest, 67, 101, 259
endometrial cancer, 23, 204,
    226
endometrium, 23, 84-85, 205
energy. *See* postmenopausal
    zest
Esalen Institute conference,
    262-65
Esselstyn, Caldwell B., Jr.,
    191-92
Estraderm patch, 129, 160,
    205-06
estrogen
  benefits vs risks, 211
  body's production of, 14,
    93
  and brain function, xix,
    43, 85, 135-37, 139-44
  and breast cancer, 175,
    184-85, 186, 188-93, 225

and depression, 97-98,
    108, 137
designer (SERMS), xix,
    224-26
and endometrial cancer,
    23
in fat intake, 191-92
and gender differences, 57-
    58
and heart disease
    prevention, 42-43, 91,
    172
loss of, 15, 22, 23, 34, 42-
    43, 61, 90, 122, 139-44,
    167
in oral contraceptives, 93,
    190, 191
and osteoporosis
    prevention, 42, 48, 156,
    180, 181-82, 225
plant, 88, 163, 200-01,
    227, 249
regimens of prescription,
    213
and sexual response, 24,
    33-34, 115, 122
and vaginal lubrication,
    126
see also hormone
    replacement therapy
Ettinger, Bruce, 181, 222
Evista, 224-25
exercise, 10, 71, 114, 154,
    160, 166, 218-19, 249,
    272
  for heart disease
    prevention, 175-76
  for osteoporosis
    prevention, 180-81

facial hair, 124
fallopian tube, 14

family history, 23, 114, 177, 184, 187-88, 209, 210, 236, 271

Family Medical Leave Act (FMLA), 75

fat, body, 44, 153-54, 191, 217

fat, dietary, 163, 175, 191-92, 219

fatigue, 6, 21, 24, 95

FDA. *See* Food and Drug Administration

fertility
    with donor egg, 110
    loss of, 41-42, 101

fertility drugs, 15, 191, 215

fibroids, 241-42, 251-53

Fillit, Howard, 97

Finch, Caleb, 145

First Wives Club, 11-12

Fisher, Helen E., 58-59

Fisher, June, 72, 74, 75

Flint, Marcha, 248

folic acid, 173

Food and Drug Administration (FDA), 26, 166, 202, 205, 226, 227

Fosamax, 225

Frank, Lawrence, 57, 61

Fretts, Ruth, 109

Freud, Sigmund, 94

Friedan, Betty, 208-09

Frye, Suzanne, 92

FSH (follicle-stimulating hormone), 105, 229

Gallup survey, 9, 129, 131

Galsworthy, Theresa, 153-54

gamma-linolenic acid, 163

Gandhi, Indira, 62

gardening, 272

gender differences, hormones in, 56-59, 63

generativity, 267-68

Gilbar, Annie, 29

ginseng, 88

Glickman, Steven, 57

Goldman, Lee, 172

Graham, Effie, 47, 130-31

Grandmother Hypothesis, 76-77

Greer, Germaine, 117, 121

Grifo, Jamie, xxv

Group Four, 262

Guber, Lynda, 28-29, 30

gynecologists
    attitude to menopausal women, 235-37
    female vs male, 22-23, 236
    and hysterectomy, 238, 239, 240-41, 252

Hadza, 76-77

Harvard Medical School, 96, 98

Hawkes, Kristen, 76, 77

Hawn, Goldie, 11-12

HDL cholesterol, 91, 173, 174, 225

health
    active participation in, 22-23, 229-30, 233-34, 242
    and biannual exams, 273
    holistic approach to, 33
    and hormonal change, 42-43, 91-92
    during perimenopause, 90-93
    self-valuing approach to, 9-10
    see also specific conditions

health insurance, 24
Healy, Bernadine, 174, 235
heart disease, 9, 10, 34, 49, 92
    and blood vessel change, 91
    and cholesterol, 173-74
    and estrogen, 42-43, 91, 172, 174-75, 199
    family history of, 210
    reducing exposure to, 173, 175-76, 192
    research on men, 242
    women's risk of, 169, 170-73, 184, 188-89
heart palpitations, 34, 82
Helen Hayes Bone Center, 98-99, 181
Henderson, Brian, 206, 209
Henderson, Victor, 143
herbal remedies, 71, 88, 160, 161-62, 166-67, 272
hip fractures, 173, 179
hippocampus, 136
holistic approach, 23, 33, 34-35
homeopathic remedies, 10, 88, 162-63
hormone replacement therapy (HRT), 17, 18, 22, 116
    and Alzheimer's disease, 143
    benefits of, 143, 174-75, 181-82, 184, 185-86, 189, 193, 199, 200, 211-12
    for breast cancer victims, 206, 245-46
    cessation of, 24-25, 117-18, 220-21, 226, 271-72
    combined hormones in, 23-24, 25, 26, 27, 124-25, 201-06, 213
    continuous, 26
    customized approach to, xx-xxi, 26, 27
    deciding on, 33-36, 140, 157-58, 184, 188-89, 197-99, 209-15, 228-30
    duration of, 184, 186, 220-21
    fear and guilt about, 33, 36
    increase in use, 27
    for men, 54-55
    natural compounds in, 201-03
    during perimenopause, 92-93
    and progesterone-sensitivity, 226-27
    reduction in dosage, 222, 271, 272
    regimens of prescription, 201, 213
    risks of, 23-24, 157-58, 160, 168-69, 184-85, 186, 188-89, 192-93, 211-12, 215
    SERMS (selective estrogen receptor modulators), xix, 224-26
    side effects of, 16, 24, 25, 211-12
    testosterone preparations in, 124-25
    transdermal patch method of, 129, 160, 205-06
    and weight gain, 16, 216-18
    see also estrogen; progesterone

hormones, 5-6, 15
  estrogen/testosterone ratio, 61
  and gender differences, 56-59, 63
  male, 56, 57, 58, 60-61, 62
  thyroid, 54-55
  see also hormone replacement therapy; *specific hormones*
hot flashes, xxii, 4-5, 16, 20-21, 25, 47, 52, 93, 108, 180, 183, 197
  natural remedies for, 163, 249
  in workplace, 75-76, 82
HRT. *See* hormone replacement therapy
Hurwich, Cecelia, 265
hypothalamus, 43, 164-65
hysterectomy, 68, 83
  and depression, 102-03
  elective, 238-39
  incidence of, 18, 238
  male response to, 130
  menopausal symptoms after, 140, 144, 221, 239
  and osteoporosis risk, 240
  ovary removal in, 19, 139-40, 239-40, 252-53
  partial, 18-19
  and sexual response, 123, 124-25, 240
  unnecessary, 240-42, 251-53
hysteroscopy, 241

Ichinose, Aloma, 35
identity crisis, 101-02
incontinence, urge, 91

insomnia. *See* sleeplessness
Ireland, Patricia, 142
irritability, 95, 96-97, 129

Japan, menopausal women in, 249-50
Journal of the National Cancer Institute, 192
Judd, Howard, 61, 123, 240

Kennedy, John, 54
kidneys, 162
Kingsberg, Sheryl, 122
Krim, Mathilde, 236-37
Kronenberg, Fredi, 235
Kuller, Lewis, 178, 192

Lancet, The, 249
Lane, Joseph, 181-82
Lavin, Linda, 11
Lawrence, Alice, 96-97
LDL cholesterol, 91, 174, 225
Ledger, William J., xxv
Leisure World Study, 209
Leventhal, Jeanne L., 103, 226
LH (lutenizing hormone), 105, 229
licorice, 88
life cycle, xvii, 7-8, 10
life expectancy, 8, 109, 143, 185, 209, 250
Life Force (Weldon), 116-17
Lindsay, Robert, xxv, 52, 90, 98-99, 174, 181, 209
Lock, Margaret, 249
Lue, Tom, 141-42
lumpectomy, 245

McEwen, Bruce, 136-37, 141
McGrath, Ellen, 39-41, 85, 102

McKinlay, Sonja and John, 96, 98
McNally, Kate, 244-45
Madison Pharmacy, 203n
malaise, 95-97, 98
male hormone. *See* testosterone
male menopause, 60-61, 141-42
mammogram, 24, 140, 245, 273
manlessness, 117, 121
Mansfield, Phyllis, 85-86
Manton, Kenneth, 8
Maslow, Abraham, 44
Massachusetts Women's Health Study, 96, 103, 241
Matera, Cristina, 26
Mead, Margaret, 13, 17, 62, 268
Medicare Bone Mass Measurement Coverage bill, 182
meditation, 88, 164, 165, 176, 180, 272, 278
Meir, Golda, 62
memory, xix, 40, 43, 70, 82, 97
  and estrogen loss, 135-39, 140-44
  natural boosters of, 147-49
men
  attitude toward menopausal women, 32-33, 68, 115, 128-31
  on hormone replacement therapy, 54-55
  and hysterectomy, 130
  menopause of, 60-61, 141-42, 264

and menstrual taboo, 128-29
menopausal symptoms, xi-xii, xviii, 40
  absence of, 44, 71, 153-54, 249
  cultural differences in, 249-50
  embarrassment caused by, 4-5, 91, 114-15, 183
  after hysterectomy, 140, 144, 221, 239
  neurological basis for, 52, 135-37, 246
  onset of, 4, 16-18, 20-21, 114, 155-56
  in perimenopause, 81-82, 114-15
  of plump vs thin women, 44, 153-54
  severity of, 26-27
  stress-related, 104-06
  in workplace, 69-70, 75-76, 82, 111, 135-36
  see also specific symptoms
menopausal women
  African-American, 250-53, 260
  family responsibilities of, 68, 101, 102, 104-05, 107, 247, 258, 263-64
  and generational change, xvi-xvii, 46-49
  healing gifts of, 267-68
  identity crisis of, 101-02
  information needs of, xii-xiv, xvi, 28-30, 34-35, 44, 87
  life expectancy of, 8, 143, 185, 209, 250
  loss of control, 155-58
  loss of fertility, 41-42

medical neglect of, 16, 22, 85, 172, 233-34, 242-43. *See also* doctors; gynecologists
men's attitudes toward, 32-33, 68, 115, 128-31
in popular culture, 11-12
in population, xv
women's attitudes toward, 6-7, 73-74, 111
in workplace. *See* workplace, menopausal women in
zest and energy of, 5, 13, 17, 61-63, 67, 76-77, 100-01, 102, 145, 161, 250, 257-74
see also menopausal symptoms; menopause
menopause
age at onset, xvii-xviii, 14-17, 83, 85
conspiracy of silence about, xiv, 3-7, 28
defined, 12, 45, 83
delaying of, 17, 109
denial of, xiv-xv, xi-xii, 31, 34-35, 37, 40-41, 43-44, 73-74, 96, 154, 159
fear of, xii, 7, 10-11, 29-30, 31-32, 36-38, 51, 86
historical attitudes toward, 50-53
ignorance and misinformation about, xv-xvi, 5, 7, 9, 28-30
individual nature of, xx-xxi, 44-45
male, 60-61, 141-42, 264
management of, 10, 45, 53, 71, 159-67, 175-76, 200-01. *See also*

health; hormone replacement therapy
mothers' experience of, 46-49, 104
natural vs medicalized, 117, 159-67, 198, 208-09
normalcy of, 10, 42
phases of, 12-13, 81
planning for, xix-xx, 210, 228-30, 264-65
politics of, xvi
positive aspects of, 67, 76-77, 257-74
postmenopausal period, 13, 95, 96, 100-03, 257-74
premature, 6, 15, 18-19, 83, 85, 106, 108
as rite of passage, 277-79
surgical. *See* hysterectomy
temporary, 104-06, 221
see also menopausal symptoms; menopausal women; perimenopause
menopause clinics, 15, 123
menopause moms, 107-10
menophobia, 6
menstrual taboo, 128-29
menstruation, 8, 10, 15
cessation of, 12, 14-15, 17, 81, 83
heavy, 85, 93, 241, 242, 244-45, 252
hormonal stimulation in, 190-91
irregular, 84-85, 93, 95
medical terminology for, 242-43
onset of, 44, 191
as polluting and dangerous, 128-29

Miccuci, Mary, 34-35
middle age. *See* aging
migraines, 25, 82, 155, 156
Mitchell, Joni, 39
Monaghan, Mona, 138
mood swings, 3, 6, 23, 82,
 94, 95, 96-97, 98, 103,
 129, 137, 246
motherhood, menopausal,
 107-10
mothers' experience of
 menopause, 46-49, 104

Nachtigall, Lila, 15, 70,
 123
Naftolin, Frederick, 136
National Black Women's
 Health Project, 251
National Institutes of
 Health, 91, 202, 242
National Osteoporosis
 Foundation, 90-91, 179
National Women's Political
 Caucus, 263
Nelson, Nita, 198-99
"nervous breakdown," 47, 95
Neugarten, Bernice, 260
New England Journal of
 Medicine, 180
New Lives for Old (Mead),
 268
*New Passages: Mapping Your
 Life Across Time*
 (Sheehy), xvii, 100
New York Menopause
 Research Foundation,
 xxiv-xxv
night sweats, 25, 31, 52, 82,
 114-15, 163
Nin, Anaïs, 53
Notelovitz, Morris, 94
Nurses' Health Study, 172,
 173, 174, 185, 214, 219

nutrition. *See* diet; herbal
 remedies; vitamin
 therapy

oophorectomy. *See* ovaries,
 removal of
Oprah, xv
oral contraceptives, 93, 190,
 191, 215
Osborne, Michael, xxiv, xxv-
 xxvi, 185, 189
osteoporosis (bone loss), 9,
 10, 34, 36, 42, 92, 113-
 14, 154, 167
 and estrogen, 42, 48, 156,
 181-82, 225
 family history of, 23, 114,
 177, 184, 209, 271
 after hysterectomy, 240
 preventive measures for,
 179-81
 risk factors for, 178-79
 and tamoxifen, 206-07
 timetable of, 90-91, 177-
 78
ovarian cancer, 207
ovarian cysts, 85
ovarian failure, 83, 106, 243
ovarian fulfillment, 243
ovaries, 14, 15, 123, 205
 removal of, 19, 139-40,
 239-40, 252-53
 testosterone production of,
 240
overweight, 44, 153-54, 191,
 214, 215, 216-18
ovulation, 14, 84

Pap smear, 140, 244
PEPI (Postmenopausal
 Estrogen/Progestin
 Intervention) trial, 174-
 75, 201-02, 217

Perfect Health (Chopra), 164
perimenopause, xi-xii, xviii,
    12, 81-131, 210, 239
  depression during, 94-99,
    100, 103
  health concerns of, 23, 90-
    92
  management of, 87-89, 92-
    93
  motherhood during, 107-
    10
  sexual response in, 112-13
  signs and symptoms of,
    23, 81-86, 114-15, 241
  and stress, 104-06, 221
  physical appearance, 4, 7,
    16, 31-32, 36-37, 101,
    113, 154, 156, 250, 251
physical examination, 22,
    234
Pilate, Pamela, 252-53
PMS, 103, 109, 210
Poehlman, Eric, 217
Poitier, Joanna, 29, 31, 33
Pollard, Eve, 43, 121
postmenopausal period, 13,
    95, 96, 100-03, 257-74
postmenopausal zest, 13, 17,
    61-62, 102, 269
postpartum depression, 108
pregnancy, 190, 191
  blood vessels in, 91
  delayed, 109-10
  and early menopause, 108
Premarin, 24, 27, 36, 88,
    206, 209
Prempro, 27
primrose oil, 163
progesterone, 23n, 25, 84,
    174
  benefits vs risks, 212
  low-dose, 201

  natural micronized, 202-
    03
  regimens of prescription,
    213
  sensitivity to, 226-27
  and weight gain, 218
progestin, 23-24
Provera, 24, 25
puberty, 21-22, 82-83
Pugh, Clementine, 251

Quindlen, Anna, xvi

raloxifene, 224, 225-26
Ramey, Estelle, 91, 113, 125,
    174
Rancho La Puerta, 163
relaxation techniques, 88,
    164, 165, 176
REM sleep, 98-99
Reno, Janet, 62
Replens, 226
Resilard, Tanya, 130
Rimm, Eric, 173
Room for Two, 11
Roosevelt, Eleanor, 62
Rose, David, 192
Royal Jelly, 88, 272

Sand, Gayle, 113-15, 126-
    27
Sand, George, 51-53
Second Adulthood, 7-8, 10,
    76, 87, 258, 265, 267
self-concept/self-esteem, 101-
    02, 250, 251, 274
SERMS (selective estrogen
    receptor modulators),
    xix, 224-26
sexual response
  and estrogen, 24, 33-34,
    115, 117, 122

sexual response *(cont.)*
  and genital discomfort,
    10, 43, 91, 92, 116, 122,
    126-27, 167
  and hysterectomy, 123,
    124-25, 240
  loss of, 21-22, 98, 102,
    113, 115, 117-18, 120-
    21
  and male menopause, 60-
    61, 141
  rekindled, 24, 112-13,
    119-20, 124, 131, 262,
    266
  and testosterone, 122,
    124-25, 240
Sherwin, Barbara, 123, 124,
  140-41, 144
Siiteri, Pentti, 60
Silent Passage, The (Sheehy),
  xiv, xx, xxiv, 18, 44
Singer, Isaac Bashevis, 56
Singha, Shyam S., xxvi, 162-
  63
Sixth International Congress
  on the Menopause, 249
skin
  and diet, 113
  dryness of, 16, 43
  itchy, 82
sleeplessness, 3, 15, 25, 43,
  47, 82, 88, 98-99, 106,
  180
Smith, Lynn, 37
smoking, 22, 166, 173, 175,
  178, 214
sonograms, 205, 273
soy milk, 89
Specht, Lisa, 31
Stampfer, Meir, 172
Stanton, Elizabeth Cady, 274
Steinem, Gloria, 120

Stevenson, Elizabeth, 269
Strang Cancer Prevention
  Center, xxiv, 185, 189
stress, 96
  and heart disease, 176
  premenstrual, 103
  reduction, 160, 162, 164,
    176
  and temporary
    menopause, 104-06, 221
  work-related, 39-40, 246
support group, 99
symptoms. *See* menopausal
  symptoms

Tai Chi, 180-81
tamoxifen, 206-07, 245-46
testosterone, 116
  and aggressiveness, 62
  benefits vs risks, 212
  and gender differences, 56,
    57, 58
  and male menopause, 60-
    61
  and ovaries, 240
  in postmenopausal
    women, 61-62, 123-24
  and sexual response, 122,
    124-25, 240
  testing for levels of, 125
Thatcher, Margaret, 62
Three Guineas (Woolf), 53
thyroid hormone, 54-55
tofu, 89, 163
Trabulus, Joyce Bogart, 42

ultrasound, 205, 207
urinary infections, 126
urination, 91-92, 126
uterine cancer, 34, 173, 204-
  05, 246
uterus, 18, 91, 240-41, 242

see also hysterectomy
Utian, Wulf, 225-26

vagina
    atrophy of, 10, 43, 92,
        122, 167
    dryness of, 91, 116, 122,
        126, 127, 140, 163, 167,
        183
    lubrication of, 126-27, 226
    sonograms of, 273
Victorian Women, 51
vitamin therapy, 88, 147-48,
    159, 163, 173, 273

walking, 166, 176, 180
Wallace, Marcia, 107-08
Wallen, Kim, 50, 190-91
Wallis, Lila A., 220, 221
Warga, Claire, 142
Warren, Leslie Ann, 31-33
weight
    effect on menopause
        symptoms, 44, 153-54
    gain, 16, 191, 214, 216-18
    loss, 105, 113, 154, 182,
        218
Weldon, Fay, 9, 116-17
well-being, postmenopausal,
    102
Whitehead, Malcolm, xxvi,
    187, 199
Willett, Walter, 185, 186,
    214
Woman as Healer
    (Achterberg), 267
Women and Depression, 102

Women's Health Initiative,
    xvi, 204, 216, 235
Women's International
    Pharmacy, 203n
Woods, Harriet, 263
Woolf, Virginia, 53
workplace, menopausal
    women in, xviii-xix, 97,
        111
    in command positions, 62,
        67, 70-71
    communication about
        health issues, 68, 72-75
    co-workers' attitude
        toward, 73-74
    legal protection for, 75
    and memory lapses, 135-
        36, 138-39
    numbers of, 69
    postmenopausal zest of,
        62-63
    and stress, 39-40, 246
    and symptom
        management, 69-70, 75-
        76, 82
    value as employees, 76
Wyeth Ayerst, 226, 227

Yalom, Marilyn, 51
yams, 163, 202
yoga, 88, 164, 176, 272

Zackson, David, xxvi, 178,
    179
Zacur, Howard, xviii, 83, 92
Zand, Janet, 167